The Healing
REVOLUTION

Eight Essentials to Awaken
Abundant Life, Naturally

Dr. Frank King

Healing Revolution Press, LLC

D1021541

*The Healing Revolution; Eight Essentials
to Awaken Abundant Life, Naturally*
By Frank J. King, Jr.

Copyright © 2014 Healing Revolution Press LLC

First published in the USA in 2013 by
Healing Revolution Press LLC
150 Westside Dr.
Asheville, NC 28806
828-255-0201
healingrevolutionllc@gmail.com

ISBN: 978-0-9894369-0-8 (print edition)
ISBN: 978-0-9894369-1-5 (digital edition)
Library of Congress Control Number: 2013912545

1. Health & Fitness / General. 2. Health & Fitness /
Alternative Therapies. 3. Health & Fitness / Healing. 4.
Health & Fitness / Healthy Living. I. King, Frank J. II. Title.

Printed in the United States.

*The information in this book is for educational purposes
only. It is not intended to replace the advice of a physician
or medical practitioner. See your healthcare provider before
trying any health technique or suggestion in this book.*

ACKNOWLEDGEMENTS

This book, *The Healing Revolution: Eight Essentials to Awaken Abundant Life, Naturally*, is the first in a series of *The Healing Revolution* books. It represents the fulfillment of a dream that was planted in my heart in the early 1970s. I always say that it takes a team to fulfill a dream, and these pages prove that's true.

I would like to express my deepest gratitude to my wife, Suzie, the great discerner, my encourager and inspirer. You have brought me more joy and beauty than I can ever describe.

Thanks also go to my children Frankie, Nathan and Bella, who have offered wisdom and insights well beyond their age. You have enriched my life in so many ways.

An amazing team of King Bio co-workers accompanied me on this journey. I don't know what I would do without my "angels" and all the research and experience they have contributed to this healing message.

Finally, I must acknowledge every one of my patients who – since the late 1970s – have taught me more than I could have learned from hundreds of books or educational courses. You have led me to priceless healing discoveries. Thank you for allowing me to share your stories in these pages.

The Healing Revolution is not only a series of books, it is also a 'self-health' movement – a journey that we are embarking on together. This journey results in health empowerment for everyone. Through The Healing Revolution® I will freely share, through videos, podcasts, speaking engagements, and online, the most effective tools and healing techniques that can help people take back their health. I'm proud to co-discover new hope, health and wholeness with all of you by my side.

ENDORSEMENTS

"Dr. King's vibrant prescription for health is a refreshing alternative to placing your trust in a bottle of pills and an ailing healthcare system. You can take responsibility for your health and well-being. You can live long and well by harnessing the healing power of nature, and *The Healing Revolution* tells you how."
— Dr. Hyla Cass, MD, author of *8 Weeks to Vibrant Health*

"Dr. Frank King teaches us not only to live long – 120 years is the goal – but also to live well. His optimistic attitude and natural techniques are life-saving for those who might feel they are barely hanging by a thread. Victims can become victors in *The Healing Revolution!*"
— Dr. Steven B. Ross, DC, DAAPM, FASBE; President and Co-founder of the Institute For Integrative Medicine, LLC

"In *The Healing Revolution*, Frank King illuminates a natural path to abundant life through sensible choices. I truly hope that this book is "the shot heard 'round the world" - the catalyst to a revolution that will bring health and healing to many people."
— Brenda Watson, "Diva of Digestion," author of New York Times Bestseller *The Fiber 35 Diet*

"Dr. Frank King is one-in-a-million. With a compassionate hand, he reaches out to those who are sick, tired, old, feeling helpless and even facing 'incurable' diseases. If you are suffering and frustrated, then *The Healing Revolution* is what you need. It is time to get back control of your health and Dr. King's revolutionary vision for a long, whole and healthy life is the answer. This book is a must-read."
— Dr. Fabrizio Mancini, President Emeritus of Parker University and bestselling author of *The Power of Self-Healing*

"Dr. Frank King triumphantly announces *The Healing Revolution*, bringing the power to heal back where it belongs: into the hands of the people! The Eight Essentials of Life are intensely practical, with commonsense dietary, fitness and lifestyle tips and techniques that will truly transform lives. Dr. King's passion shines as bright as "Dr. Sunshine," so be illuminated as you put these eight healing essentials into practice."
— Robert Scott Bell, D.A. Hom., host of The Robert Scott Bell Show

"*The Healing Revolution* is so simple, yet all-encompassing, with timeless, natural suggestions to awaken the human, genetic potential for a long, healthy and vibrant life. I offer hearty thanks to Dr. Frank King for sounding the call for a revolution."

– Dr. Sherrill Sellman, ND, author of *Hormone Heresy: What Women MUST Know About Their Hormones*

"Dr. Frank King sees an end to the healthcare crisis by way of *The Healing Revolution*. I heartily embrace the picture he paints of a vibrant life lived well into the second century. He offers natural, life-breathing choices for exasperated people who desperately wish to avoid the killing plagues of the 21st century."

– Dr. Garry F. Gordon, MD, DO; President of the Gordon Research Institute

---

"Optimal health is more than just the right foods; it includes lifestyle factors like sleep, exercise, finding a purpose bigger than yourself and positive relationships. In his new book *The Healing Revolution*, Dr. Frank King puts the puzzle pieces together with the Eight Essentials that provide a comprehensive, easy-to-apply approach to health, healing, and a newfound joy and vitality to life. This book can totally transform your health and your life."

– JJ Virgin, CNS, CHFS, author of *The Virgin Diet*

"Dr. King's *The Healing Revolution* pays homage to the adage, 'Sound mind, healthy body.' No one is exempt from the principles outlined in this book. Truly empowering."

– Dr. Brett Osborn, DO: Neurosurgeon

"Dr. King has created *The Healing Revolution*. It is a book you truly need in your library."

– Dr. Earl Mindell, RPh, PhD, author of *The New Vitamin Bible, Herb Bible* and *Prescription Alternatives*

CONTENTS

WHY ARE YOU READING THIS?

Why are you reading this? Maybe you "just happened" to pick this book up, but I believe it's more than a chance occurrence.

I believe this is a quantum leap opportunity on your personal journey to health, happiness, wholeness and a total-life makeover. Welcome to the HEALING REVOLUTION!

It is my desire that you discover your amazing life potential in the pages to come. You will learn how we are all people destined for wonderful opportunities and greater lives, yet we have undersold ourselves. We are like thoroughbred horses who are locked inside a dark and moldy shed. I don't know about you, but I long to breathe the fresh air and run free through grassy meadows in the open sunshine!

In the coming chapters, I will tell you about the oldest, healthiest and happiest people on earth, living in what are known as the "Blue Zones." Some of these folks who were born before the sinking of the Titanic in 1912 are still caring for their farms, tending sheep on rocky hillsides, loving their spouses and escaping the popular ailments that kill so many people today. I will show you how science has decoded the secrets residing in your genes that can enable you to live a healthy, happy and productive life beyond 100 years.

Unfortunately most of us live in a "polluted gray zone" where we over-stress, under-exercise and super-size ourselves into an early grave. I'm thinking of many people I know who – perhaps like you – desire greater joy, excellent health and a more fulfilling life. I have stood with countless men, women and children at this critical crossroads as they struggled to leave bad habits and poor lifestyle choices behind. Thankfully many discovered their healing potential within, while others remained or even died at the crossroads.

> *The choice of which road to take is up to the individual. He alone can decide whether he wants to reach a dead end or live a healthy lifestyle for a long, healthy, happy, active life.*
>
> **– Dr. Paul C. Bragg, Health Movement Pioneer**

I remember standing at that intersection of life and death with a woman named Julie.[1] "I feel so tired and helpless," she confessed with tears in her eyes. "I constantly struggle with my weight and my health. I know I should change, but I can't. I get so depressed. My life is a sinking spiral and I can't stop sliding down."

My words to Julie are also my words to you. "Don't be discouraged. Your mind, body and spirit are created for an awesome purpose. You can be whole and healthy. Don't let avoidable health problems force you to say goodbye to happiness, freedom, mental clarity and creative work. You have the power and potential within you *to live a long and fulfilling life*. You *can* become whole if you don't give up. Do you believe that's true?"

Let me stress that this is not a program of bucking up, gritting your teeth and forcibly changing lifestyle habits. If it was, I would be setting you up for another failed diet or exercise program. Instead, I will give you powerful life-transforming tools that have been tested and proven to be effective by so many people just like you.

So why are you reading this? It is no accident that you have come to the crossroads. This is the first day of your Healing Revolution. Your joy-filled destiny lies around the next corner. You can succeed, just like many people who have walked this path before you.

> *A hundred years is securely established as the human potential.*
>
> **– Dr. Walter Bortz II of Stanford University, author of *Roadmap to 100***

Now what do you say? Shall we start a revolution?

Yes! Let's get started!

Tell us about your journey to health and wholeness at www.DrFrankKing.com, where you will find more helpful information about the Healing Revolution.

---

1   Some of the names in this book have been changed to respect people's privacy.

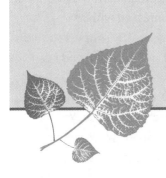

MY CROSSROADS

*It matters not what your present age is or
what your physical condition. If you obey
nature's laws, you can be born again.*

– Dr. Paul C. Bragg

I was in college and – like most students – accustomed to pinching myself during sleepy lectures. Perhaps that's one reason why Dr. Paul Bragg's presentation left me thunderstruck and speechless. I was astounded not so much by the elderly man's spoken words as by his physical posture.

Unbelievable, I thought. *He is actually standing on his head!*

At 80 years of age, Paul Bragg lectured upside-down with more poise and grace than many people I knew who were accustomed to speaking the ordinary way up. I glanced at my watch.

He's been up for nearly ten minutes. This guy is amazing!

With his gray-haired dome planted in the carpet, Paul Bragg lectured as nonchalantly as if he were reclining in an easy chair. I can't remember everything he said that day, but I will never forget his delivery. Every word was so positive, vibrant, uplifting and life-enhancing.

Paul Bragg eventually righted his world view, giving me a clearer picture of an amazing man. To me, he was a paradox of youthful vigor in a vintage body. I took a guess at his date of birth, and was amazed to know that Paul Bragg would have been about seven years old when the Wright Flyer soared over Kitty Hawk. Now here he was still acting like a kid, though the world had changed dramatically all around him. I studied his statuesque features: his sturdy arms; his bronze, youthful skin; his bright smile; and the mischievous sparkle in his eyes. To me, it was as if a sculpted Greek deity had taken breath and stepped off a granite pedestal to walk among us. Every word he spoke was life to me.

He attributed his health to decades of right living. To this day, Paul Bragg is known as a patriarch of the health movement in America. His passion for natural living totally transformed many people's lives including Jack LaLanne, the "godfather of fitness."

That lecture was my epiphany. It was as if the Rocky Theme Song thundered in my head (even though Sylvester Stallone was was probably still in high school). I was struck with amazement. I walked away absolutely transformed, with a new portrait of abundant life etched in my soul. Until then, "old age" had conjured in my mind the crippled image of a frail old man or woman leaning on a cane. Paul Bragg offered an alluring alternative: the picture of a spirited old rascal standing on his head. Moreover, Paul said that I could actually choose the quality of my life. *I was the architect rather than the victim of my destiny.*

Sadly, I heard that Paul Bragg died a year or two after I'd seen him. His family reported that a surfing accident caused complications that contributed to his "early" demise. I was aghast when I heard the news.

A surfing accident!

I had never heard of anyone surfing in their 80s. This outlandish man was smashing all my stereotypes.

Paul Bragg showed me my personal crossroads. For the first time in my life, I saw that I could choose what quality of life I wanted to live. Down one road I saw a frail old man with a cane. Down a second road I saw a man living life to the fullest, outrunning the devil to the end of the dock and diving into the water with a hearty laugh. I looked hard and saw that the faces of the men on both roads were identical.

It's me, I observed. *The faces are mine. The choice is mine.*

This is where I choose my destiny.

I didn't hesitate for one second. That day I set off running down the road to health and wholeness. I have never turned back. A brand new picture captured my attention. It was an exciting, invigorating image of me. In that picture I am living long and living well with the ones I love.

Who knows? Maybe I will meet my Maker at 110 while riding a huge wave off the coast of Australia.

What a way to go!

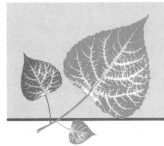

THE REVOLUTION STARTS HERE

Every man is the builder of a temple called his body. We are all sculptors and painters and our material is our own flesh, blood and bones.

– Henry David Thoreau

> *It is health that is real wealth and not pieces of gold and silver.*
>
> **– Mahatma Gandhi**

Jane and John are within spitting distance of a critical crossroads, although they are sadly mired in The Great Rut. They don't have much to look forward to in this rut, either good or bad, but they're making the best of it. The drudgery of life barely leaves them enough energy to take nourishment in front of the tube each night. But they try not to complain because the bills get paid – well, mostly. As for health, sure Jane and John have their ups and downs – who doesn't? But they hope to retire at 65. Then they plan to spend time with the grandkids and maybe travel a little. After that ... well, they don't talk much about "after that." If they follow their family pattern, they're not likely to live long. That's just how life goes in The Great Rut.

Like each one of us, Jane and John are experiencing the best and the worst of the 21st century. Jane and John are quick to buy the latest products that shape their lives, while being slow to recognize the negative side effects upon long-term health and happiness. In fact, many of the conveniences that Jane and John presume to be the rewards of the modern world – when taken together – are wreaking havoc upon their quality of life.

Modern medicine and machines may extend Jane and John's life a few months or years, but the *questionable quality* of that life makes old age undesirable – and that's an understatement. This is the price of life in the 21st century. It's a sickly life that we have created with our dollars and our choices. We are patronizing our own demise.

The *good news* is that we can experience the best of both worlds. We can enjoy the best of the 21st century, while embracing the life-giving aspects of a healthy lifestyle that many people today have forgotten. We have the incredible potential to live longer, healthier lives than our great-grandparents thought possible. We are unlikely to die from the common plagues and ailments that devastated previous generations. The chances of getting eaten by wild animals are slim. We have access to good dentists, urgent care, healthy foods, natural medicines and more knowledge than ever about healthy living. Our generation is unique in that we can expect to live both healthy and comfortable lives – well beyond 100 years of age – but only if we make the right choices.

Unfortunately, Jane and John are wasting away in The Great Rut of modernity, not having heard about healthy choices. Worst of all, Jane and John do not even realize that anything is wrong. They don't know that they are, in truth, people of unfulfilled destiny, created for a joy-filled purpose far greater than they can imagine.

It makes me want to shout, "We desperately need a Healing Revolution!"

SONYA'S AWAKENING

I'm reminded of a woman named Sonya who hobbled into my office one day. She was bent over and fatigued, which surprised me since she was an attractive young woman in her twenties. Her brow was furrowed and her lips puckered.

The curtain has closed on her life, I thought. *She's withdrawn. Her fuel tank is on empty. She's obviously in pain. She looks as if she's a prisoner of her own body.*

Sonya told me about the sinus and intestinal issues that plagued her. She was at the end of her rope, having tried several doctors, drugs and remedies. All of her healthcare expenses were covered by the state, and she had a shelf full of free prescription drugs, but her quality of life sank lower each day. Having little hope and nothing to lose, she decided to give our holistic, naturopathic approach a try. So we counseled her to make some simple changes in her diet and lifestyle, which she readily accepted.

In the following weeks, Sonya experienced quick relief from her painful symptoms. Under her doctor's care, she quit her prescription drugs. She ate better and exercised. She drank more water and got more sleep. She made positive changes in the Eight Essential areas of health. She even attended some of my health lectures and made new friends while she was there. That was so important, since unlike her old friends who reinforced a victim-mentality, these new companions encouraged her with a more positive outlook on life.

Gradually Sonya's whole demeanor brightened. Her energy and enthusiasm rocketed to the sky. Like so many other people I've known, her changes were nothing short of miraculous. Sonya literally became a new person. Her eyes began to brighten. She stood straighter, displaying confidence and hope. She was excited about her new lifestyle. It was as if she had burst from an early grave and was born again.

Most importantly, Sonya came to believe that the power to heal was within her, and she was determined to awaken that healing power.

The last time I saw Sonya, she was youthful and vibrant. Her smile was captivating. A new joy and happiness had taken root in her heart. Her face shone with the brilliance of the morning sun.

"Guess what, Dr. King?" Sonya asked me that day. "I'm going to college."

"That's wonderful, Sonya. I'm so proud of you!" This news was especially significant since it meant Sonya was breaking a tradition. Most of her family was unemployed and deeply rooted in the welfare system.

"I've taken an interest in advertising and marketing, Dr. King. I wrote some pretty good jingles. I think I'm a natural. So I applied for college ... and I got accepted!"

I was so happy for Sonya. She showed me how a person's health affects nearly everything in life. She broke out of The Great Rut and set off not walking, not jogging, but sprinting down the road to a better life.

YOU CAN DO IT

I am excited to begin this journey to wholeness with you, but I don't want to rush ahead too fast. First I need to make a few qualifications:

▶ *This is not a "program" just for strong-willed people.* I promise that I will not tell you to grit your teeth, quit doing bad things, start doing good things, praise yourself when you succeed, beat yourself up when you fail and spend hours each day memorizing exhaustive lists of healthy foods, products and practices. I will, however, give you some simple tools that have helped many men, women and children just like you succeed. I will show you nature's natural path to healing.

▶ *This is not another quick-fix or magic pill.* You've probably heard the claims: "This incredible new discovery will extend your life, heal your sickness, strengthen your relationships, shrink your waistline and fatten your bank account in 90 days." That kind of offer probably sounds too good to be true because it is. This is not like one of those latest fads. The Healing Revolution is intuitive and organic. It recalls the best natural, life-affirming choices that have stood the test of time. Research has consistently validated the benefits of natural medicines, naturopathic remedies, healthy lifestyles and positive attitudes. I will share stories and research going back to my first clinic in 1979, validating the need for a holistic approach encompassing all Eight Essential factors of life.

▶ *The Healing Revolution is where the best health ideas come together.* In recent years, experts have announced the benefits of many different diets, exercise routines, water-drinking programs and positive-attitude plans. There are so many competing claims that they can't possibly all be true. And yet I have found some truth in many of these programs, but not for all people, all of the time. The Healing Revolution embraces the best elements, integrating them into the Eight Essentials of life. The beauty and attraction of the Eight Essentials of life is that you get better, more comprehensive results with less time and effort than programs that single out components like mental health, physical exercise, attitudes or diet. You can't expect to help the whole person by improving just a few areas.

▶ **You can improve the quality of your life, whatever your age or condition.** Most people I have worked with do not – at the beginning – truly believe they can be healed. Maybe they've "tried everything," or they have a low self-image. Maybe their parents suffered with a similar ailment and they feel as if their own destiny lies down that same, rocky path. Many actually sabotage their own health without even knowing it. They themselves are the biggest obstacle to their own healing. If you are inclined to think these thoughts, check them at the door! Your body is designed to remain strong and healthy past 100 years of age. Whether you live for another year or for another century, your quality of life is most important. Don't settle for anything short of excellence. Choose life! When people ask me if I had a good day, I typically answer, "No. I did not have a good day. I had a great day!" You will receive wholeness to the level which you seek it.

> *First they ignore you. Then they ridicule you. And then they attack you and want to burn you. And then they build monuments to you.*
>
> *– Trade unionist Nicholas Klein (1914)*

▶ **Some of these ideas may challenge your traditional thought.** Please don't run away if some of these concepts seem strange or new to you. Healthy skepticism is a good thing. Stick around to get all your questions answered. People have always questioned what is new and different. For example, research is only beginning to grapple with the powerful bioenergetic forces connected with the human body. "I don't buy into that New Age rubbish," some people say. "I only believe what I can see, touch or measure with a machine." Who would claim that our generation has discovered all that can be known and that everything else is voodoo? Galileo Galilei faced the Inquisition because he maintained that the sun was at the center of the solar system. A world with people standing upside-down on the other side was illogical and inconceivable to most people. Where are the flat earth proponents today? Hopefully our great-grandchildren will someday say, "Do you remember flat earth medicine?"

▶ **I can help you get started on this journey, but soon you will be on your own.** If the Eight Essentials are like eight life-giving gardens, then I am the gardener and gatekeeper. I will show you the path to these gardens and then I will turn you loose on your own self-guided tour. You will not need me once you learn how to awaken and empower your own healing potential. I will share with you the Eight Essentials that you need to succeed. I will be your personal life-coach, helping you when you need it, sharing these new healing techniques to help your inner garden grow and prosper.

THE POWER TO HEAL IS WITHIN YOU

> *The greatest of follies is to sacrifice health for any other kind of happiness.*
>
> *– 19th century philosopher Arthur Schopenhauer*

Perhaps the greatest so-called "secret" is this: **THE POWER TO HEAL IS WITHIN YOU.**

Picture this scenario: a wise person discovered the secret healing power that enabled people to live long and fulfilling lives. That person went to the Highest Power in the Universe and said, "In which hidden vault shall we hide this priceless treasure so that people will not lose it?" The reply came back, "I have already hidden that power within them."

This is the essence of the Healing Revolution. This essence is the raw, potent, seductive energy of life that emanates from our hearts and souls, that binds each one of us together and to the earth.

The secret is within you.

You can live long. You can live well. You can live healthy. You can discover your potential.

The Healing Revolution starts here!

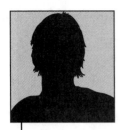

Doug's Story: Dying for Others

Doug's greatest passion was to lay his hands on sick people and pray for their healing. His life calling was to be a preacher. His whole life revolved around the church. He cared for each person as tenderly as a parent for an only child.

Pastor Doug was about 70 pounds overweight when he came to me for treatment. As with many patients, I could see that the pain he wanted me to treat was only the tip of an iceberg of problems. So I treated the obvious symptoms while looking for opportunities to help him with his larger lifestyle issues.

Doug worked too hard, slept too little, ate too much and didn't like to exercise. Throughout the months that I saw him, the lines of stress deepened on his kind and compassionate face. He was an enigma, giving his life so sacrificially for others while caring so little for himself. His body was being pummeled by his choices, unable to restore and refresh itself under the hefty heap of pressures weighing it down.

At first I talked gently to Pastor Doug, urging him to make a few small changes. I coached him to take more time away from work, to go for small walks and to eat better.

"Oh, I'm fine," he would tell me. "I'm doing the things that I enjoy. This is my life's passion. As for my health, everybody has a few aches and pains. But I'm doing God's work and God will take care of me."

In time I took a more forthright approach, preaching at the preacher. But however forcefully I coaxed, cajoled, or nagged, his answer was always the same.

"I'm doing fine."

You can imagine my shock when I heard the news from one of his church members: "Pastor Doug had a heart attack. He's ... dead."

Pastor Doug was 51-years-young when the people he loved more than himself placed his coffin in the green grass beside his beloved church.

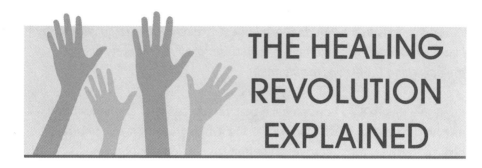

THE HEALING REVOLUTION EXPLAINED

Life doesn't get much better than when you're holed-up in an old cabin in the Allegany Mountains. When I was 13, my dad would drive our two-tone '58 Buick along the twisted Allegany River up from Oil City, Pennsylvania, then he'd set me free like a bandit. Those were days when the sun never seemed to set.

Have you ever been so excited about a day that you could hardly wait to get up? That's how each morning was in that little cabin overlooking the Allegany River. We'd gather larva from under the rocks in the river, then use them for bait while fishing from my dad's little boat with a three horsepower Johnson outboard motor. We'd climb massive boulders or skip stones so many times you'd think they were floating ducks.

A massive oak tree grew at the top of a steep bank that dropped 20 feet to the river's edge. I'm not sure who tied the long rope to a limb that hung way out, but I could only reach it by leaning over the edge and hooking it with the end of a stick. I'd pull that rope over to one side of the tree and run over the cliff screaming like a banshee and holding on to save my life. The momentum would swing me in a wide arc over the river, then I'd land on the other side of the tree, my feet still running. Gosh, that was a thrill!

Nothing could stop me from packing each day full of adventure – not even the time I got a concussion when I flipped my bike upside-down over my dog Lassie, who got tangled in my tires. Strange to say, I can't even remember stopping to eat meals during the course of a normal day. I do remember waking up so hungry one night that I tiptoed in pitch darkness into the kitchen and grabbed what I thought to be a fig bar. The "tasty treat" turned out to be a bar of calamine soap. Needless to say, I spent some time leaning over the kitchen sink, washing my mouth with water while bubbles came out like soda from a shaken can of pop. You might say that was my first taste of natural medicine.

Those were the best days. All of life seemed bright and promising. Even the mishaps became things to laugh at. Everybody seems to have days like those that they cherish for the rest of their lives.

So you may ask: *What do those unbeatable days have to do with today? I barely dragged my carcass out of bed this morning. This brew in my cup is the only thing that keeps me standing.*

Know this: TODAY you can have that vibrant sense of excitement and discovery. Life is so much more rewarding when you embrace a naturally healthy lifestyle. You feel so much better. Even when troubles come, your capacity to handle the bumps in the road increases. Life need not go "downhill" month-by-month after that certain birthday you've been dreading. Life can keep getting better all the time!

The Healing Revolution is not a system of dos and don'ts. It's not a stringent health "program." Instead, the Healing Revolution is all about discovering the power of life and its potentials that are already within you. The tools for vibrant health are in your genes. They are awakened by your life-affirming choices, activated in your hands and fingertips. The Eight Essentials of life will guide you in this exciting journey to a long and happy life.

THE HEALING REVOLUTION EXPLAINED

These are the ***foundational truths*** of the Healing Revolution. Everything else builds upon these truths.

- *You are genetically designed to live a long, healthy, abundant life.*
- *The absence of disease is merely the **beginning** of abundant life. You are floating in a sea of opportunity. The Healing Revolution frees you to reach your highest potential, soaring high in the sky like an eagle.*
- *The power to heal is within you.*
- *There is no such thing as an incurable disease.*
- *You are an integrative, whole being: the health of your body, mind and spirit are intertwined.*
- *Your lifestyle choices have a significant impact upon your health and happiness.*
- *Many of today's foods, activities and lifestyle choices inhibit your body's ability to heal and restore itself.*
- *Separated from your genetic roots, you are like a polar bear struggling to survive in the desert.*

- *A natural lifestyle removes negative health inhibitors.*
- *A natural lifestyle frees the healing powers and potential within you.*
- *By making small, positive choices in all Eight Essentials of life, you accomplish more than if you make big changes in a few areas. You can work smarter, not harder. (The Eight Essentials are explained later.)*
- *Your attitude will determine your altitude. To reach the highest heights, have an open mind, a tender heart, an active will, a thicker skin and a positive attitude.*
- *Your whole being is the doctor and the healer, 24/7.*

Embedded within you is a powerful healing force. Modern life often places inhibitions upon your healing force, by the way you choose to eat, drink, sleep, relate, believe and respond to stress. If you do nothing more than remove these inhibitions, your natural life forces are freed to heal.

You can simply learn to defend, protect and awaken your whole being, the healer. You can easily learn to close the gates that allow all the scum to sleaze in and pollute your life. You are the gate-keeper, not your doctor, therapist, social worker, parent or spouse. Accept the reality that you are in charge of your destiny. Awaken your healing forces. Learn to work smarter, not harder. Learn to tap into your remarkable ability to heal.

Tune into your natural instincts, which will lead you to make healthy choices in all Eight Essentials of life. On the farm, I have seen animals who – when given the choice – instinctively know what food and nutritional choices are best. Chimpanzees in Africa chew on nasty-tasting herbs when they are feeling sick, as a natural remedy. Not all baboons in Ethiopia eat a natural de-worming fruit; only those who need it. Elephants in Kenya dig deep into a dangerous cave to mine a mineral that fulfills a sodium deficiency in their diet[2]. Animals like those are not the only creatures with amazing instincts. You and I can live healthier and happier lives if we learn to tune into the quiet voice of our forgotten instincts.

Your genetic destiny, as proven by the longest-living people of the world, is to live a healthy, happy and meaningful life into your second century. Did you know that the keys to a long and vibrant life are actually written in your genes?

---

2   *Animal Instinct*, www.theguardian.com/education/2002/jan/17/highereducation.healthandwellbeing (January 2014).

EPIGENETICS

Epigenetics is the science of how to change genetic expression by lifestyle choices, positive mental attitudes and belief systems. "Genetic expression" is the body's power to determine which genes can or cannot express themselves for or against your best health.

Therefore, you are not destined to fall prey to bad genetics. YOU are the author of your own health story. YOU are free to choose the ending to your story.

Epigenetics is an outgrowth and extension of the landmark Human Genome Project, which mapped 25,000 genes and three billion chemical base pairs in the human chromosomes. I won't be surprised if this exciting new science is proclaimed to be the most significant health-related discovery of the 21st century. The impact of epigenetics on the pond of human studies is more like a tsunami than a ripple. [3]

According to Mark Hyman, author of *NutriGenomics*, "The food you eat is actually information that 'talks' to your genes and washes over your DNA to create your state of health ... You can create either health or disease, and weight loss or weight gain. The exciting part is that we have significant control over the genetic messages that get turned on or off." [4]

---

[3]   I like the word "epigenomics," which applies globally to changes in the entire genome, embracing the entirety of hereditary information. In this section, however, I write "epigenetics" which is more commonly used in reference to changes in genetic expression due to environmental, behavior and attitudinal factors.

[4]   Mark Hyman, *NutriGenomics: How Food Talks to Your Genes to Send Messages of Health or Disease Workbook,* (Sarasota FL: Nutrigenomics Products, Inc., (2006), 11.

Epigenetics has knocked many of the old-school assumptions about genetics upside-down. The findings prove that lifestyle choices are, in many cases, more powerful than chromosomes. For you, specifically, this means:

◆ *You are not a victim of your genes, ruled by your genetic composition.*
◆ *You can improve genetic predispositions with thoughtful lifestyle choices, attitudes and beliefs.*
◆ *You are not destined to fall victim to illnesses like cancer, heart disease, or Alzheimer's just because of the genetic tendencies that run in your family.*

Dr. Ajay Goel of the Gastrointestinal Cancer Research Laboratory at Baylor Research Institute says, "Everything we do from the day we are born, everything we eat, drink and are exposed to in our environment has an indirect but strong influence on our genetics. As we age and grow, it is very natural that some of the genes tend to get turned off as a consequence of our [poor] eating habits, lack of exercise and exposure to toxic environmental stresses … Epigenetic alterations have a unique characteristic that these changes are *reversible*." [5]

This is amazing! Not one of us needs to be like Jane and John who were mentioned earlier, destined to grow sick and die young in The Great Rut of mediocrity. For many years, I have seen the principles of epigenetics at work, with even my "toughest" patients finding wholeness and freedom from their so-called genetic "destinies."

You don't have to be a victim! You can choose to live long and live well. Barring unavoidable accidents, you are the master of your health. You can choose your destiny.

This whole-person perspective embodies the spirit of the Human Being, not the Human Doing. You are not just what you eat. You are what you think, act and believe. You ARE the image that you carry about yourself. A wise man once said, "Where there is no vision, the people perish." [6] The best sports teams intuitively know this to be true, consistently rising to a higher level than those teams who are stuck with a negative self-image. Every successful sports team and business has a strategic plan for success. Do you have a life plan for success? We all need vision to rise above our circumstances.

You become what you believe, so believe until you become.

---

5   Ajay Goel as quoted in Jan McBarron, *Curcumin: The 21st Century Cure* (Brevard, NC: Take Charge Books, 2011), 12.
6   Attributed to King Solomon in *The Bible*, Proverbs 29:18.

In case you haven't noticed, I am *beyond* passionate about healthy living. My greatest joy will be, in the coming years, to hear the success stories of men and women like you whose lives have risen above mediocrity, above genetic predispositions and who have found new life, light and wholeness in the Healing Revolution.

BLUE ZONES

> *You cannot tailor-make the situations in life but you can tailor-make the attitudes to fit those situations.*
>
> *– Motivational speaker Zig Ziglar*

Demographers have identified five global "Blue Zones" where people experience fulfilling lives well beyond the 100-year milestone. Healthy lifestyle choices enable these people to overcome chronic diseases while filling their days with meaningful work and quality relationships, right up to the time of death. These people are not just "lucky" to live healthy lives to about the age of 120. They are reaping the benefits of good choices.

Dan Buettner, author of *The Blue Zones,*[7] interviewed a 102-year-old man living in the mountainous interior of the Italian island of Sardinia who tended sheep from dawn to dusk, ate small but healthy meals, took a nap at noon, drank a liter of Sardinian wine a day and socialized with his friends in the village most evenings. This gentleman's habits are typical of all long-living people in the Blue Zones.

Some of the common traits of these people include a physically active lifestyle, a sparse but healthy diet, fermented food or wine, good ties to friends and family and a sense of purpose. Although genetics plays a part in Blue Zone longevity, it's not a large part; researchers estimate that longevity is only influenced up to 20 percent by genetics. The five Blue Zone regions include Okinawa, Japan; Sardinia, Italy; Icaria, Greece; Nicoya Peninsula, Costa Rica; and a small Seventh Day Adventist community in Loma Linda, California.

It is interesting to note how ancient religious writings validate the Blue Zone findings. For example, the book of Genesis in the Bible says, "From now on [after the flood] people can expect to live 120 years." People allegedly lived much longer before the flood.[8]

---

7   Dan Buettner, *The Blue Zones* (Washington, DC: National Geographic Society, 2012).
8   *The Bible*, Genesis 6:3. Moses, who wrote most of the book of Genesis, allegedly lived to be 120 and was strong to the end.

"There is now a virtual consensus that the maximum human lifespan is around 120 years," says Walter Bortz, author of *Dare to Be 100*. "Natural life expectancy should conform to a bell-shaped curve, the extreme end of which is 120 years. If 120 is the far edge of the curve, where is the center [of life expectancy]? The answer is 100."[9] So while most people tend to think that living to the age of 100 years is extreme, it is in truth "average." We have set our expectations too low. Abundant life exceeds all expectations.

Most centenarians function quite well. Thirty-one percent manage their own self-care. Seventy-two percent get around without walkers or canes.[10] These centenarians prove our potential. These are the old folks we hope to become. Their daily routines might seem strange to us, but when you think about it, we are the strange ones. We are the ones who have abandoned the healthy choices that have sustained people for many generations. We have much to learn from our wise elders.

NATURAL HEALING ARTS

Modern people often miss two simple facts: 1) Drugs and doctors are not "healers," and 2) our bodies are healers. It's an important distinction to make.

To illustrate, imagine cutting a fresh steak down the middle. All the drugs and doctors in the world cannot make that gash heal, because the animal's life-force is absent.

> *Birthdays are good for your health. Studies have shown that people who have the most birthdays live the longest.*

The belief that "doctors heal" may seem like a subtle mistake, but it has actually led to a huge misplaced trust – a trust that should be placed in the powerful healing force within each one of us. Naturopathy and homeopathy seek to restore trust where it belongs, while not depreciating the doctor's appropriate role in facilitating the body's natural healing.

Allow me to explain "naturopathy" and "homeopathy," in case those terms are new to you:

Naturopathy is natural healthcare. Naturopathy uses nature to restore and maintain health. It seeks to activate the powerful, safe and effective

---

9   Walter Bortz, *Dare to Be 100* (New York: Palgrave Macmillan, 2010) p. 21.
10   Ibid, p. 79.

healing powers of the human body and of nature to correct imbalances and relieve suffering. The Healing Revolution is a naturopathic approach to health and wholeness.

Homeopathy is a natural system of medicine that involves administering substances in trace amounts that might cause adverse symptoms in large doses, to activate the body's self-healing abilities. Homeopathy's fundamental assertion is that "like cures like." This principle is similar to vaccinations that introduce pathogens into the body to activate the immune system, although homeopathy is much safer and has no known adverse reactions or contraindications.

When I speak to large groups of people, I often ask, "How many people have used homeopathy?" I might see 200 hands go up. Then I ask, "How many people have experienced profoundly positive results from homeopathy?" The same 200 hands go up. Finally I ask, "How many people have taken a homeopathic remedy, and nothing happened?" Then the same 200 hands go up. These remedies are extremely safe and effective; you simply must find the remedies that work best for you. Unlike conventional drugs, these remedies have no negative side effects or risks, allowing you to safely try different remedies until you find that profoundly positive result.

Homeopathy builds upon 200 years of data about the human body's response to natural substances. It comes with none of the surprises that occasionally plague conventional medicine and pharmaceuticals – as happened when doctors discovered that thalidomide caused stunted-limb birth defects, or more recently when hormone replacement therapy was linked to cancer, stroke and heart disease.

I am not an extremist and I am grateful for conventional medicine where it is appropriate, but I do advise people to use it with caution because of the high potential dangers. For example, a 2013 study of hospitals in the United States revealed that "premature deaths associated with preventable harm [by medical professionals] to patients was estimated at more than 400,000 per year."[11] That figure is astounding, making deaths by medical error the number three cause of death in America today, after cancer and heart disease.

American doctors administered more than 4,000,000,000 (4 billion) prescriptions for conventional drugs in 2011, or about 13 prescriptions for

---

11   John T. James, "A New, Evidence-based Estimate of Patient Harms Associated with Hospital Care," *Journal of Patient Safety*, September 2013, vol. 9, no. 3, 122–128.

> *A 2013 study of hospitals in the United States revealed that "premature deaths associated with preventable harm to patients was estimated at more than 400,000 per year."*

every man, woman and child.[12] When taken as directed, these prescribed drugs cause an average of 100,000 deaths each year.[13] Many or most of these drugs – which should be our last choice, not our first – are prescribed for conditions that could simply be eliminated with healthy lifestyle choices.

Whereas conventional medicine frequently suppresses symptoms (such as headaches, skin rashes or fevers), naturopathy and homeopathy seek to address the root causes. Symptoms like pain or swelling – or even emotional responses like anger or depression – are messengers of deeper human needs. They point to root causes.

Suppressing a symptom drives the problem deeper into the body. People who treat psoriasis or skin rashes with medication, for example, are prone to later develop chronic lung disorders or digestive problems, because the root issues have never been resolved. Every symptom communicates something that needs to be expressed, not suppressed.

Naturopathy is not opposed to safe and effective conventional medicine. It seeks to unleash a natural dimension that takes healthcare to a higher level. Naturopathic doctors like me help patients in these ways:

◆ *We seek holistic healing (for the whole person: mind, body and spirit), rather than treating a problem in isolation. The solutions to health problems are found within the whole person.*
◆ *We administer comprehensive Whole Health Appraisals to identify health issues, to prescribe appropriate treatment and to recommend helpful lifestyle choices.*
◆ *We seek to remove unnatural impediments to natural healing.*
◆ *We teach tools and techniques to improve health and wholeness.*
◆ *We recommend natural medicines and remedies.*
◆ *We prescribe remedies for the whole person, not just the disease, because we recognize the diverse needs of each individual.*

---

12   *Record 4.02 Billion Prescriptions In United States In 2011*, www.medicalnewstoday.com/releases/250213.php (January 2014).

13   Melody Petersen, *Our Daily Meds: How the Pharmaceutical Companies Transformed Themselves into Slick Marketing Machines and Hooked the Nation on Prescription Drugs* (New York: Picador-Macmillan, 2009).

- When appropriate, we refer people to conventional doctors for treatment.
- We empower people to take charge of their health. You are your body's best doctor.

Naturopathy, homeopathy, chiropractic, acupuncture and other natural healing arts simply free the human body, mind and spirit to do what they were designed to do, which is to heal naturally and live long and well.

> *When the patient loves his disease, how unwilling he is to allow a remedy to be applied.*
>
> **– French Tragedian Pierre Corneille**

HEALING BUDDIES HAVE HEALING HEARTS

Your healing journey will be much more successful if you have healing buddies to help and encourage you along the way. A healing buddy is someone who knows and loves you well. They are friends or family members who can be trusted with your needs. They believe in you.

The more healing buddies you have, the better, but have at least one. Share this book with your healing buddies so you'll all be "on the same page." Share your life-affirming choices with your healing buddies.

The best healing relationships are mutual, with each person encouraging the other, staying in regular communication and cycling the positive energy around for maximum results. Commit to meet regularly and to assist each other with the specific tools that will be explained.

SELF-EVALUATION

Self-evaluation is critical for tracking your journey to wholeness. Keep a journal of your personal revelations. I encourage you to take a blank sheet of paper and separate it into two columns, or use the form provided below and at the end of each chapter. On the left side, list the negative, life-destroying choices that you would like to leave behind. In the right column, include new life-affirming choices and attitudes that you would like to embrace, as well as positive choices that are already a part of your life. Later we'll do this exercise more specifically for each of the Eight Essentials. For now, focus on the most obvious and more general issues.

My Life-Destroying Choices	My Life-Affirming Choices
(e.g.: bad attitudes, not exercising, working too much, smoking)	*(e.g.: laugh and enjoy each moment, value friendships more, eat more natural foods)*
1	1
2	2
3	3
4	4
5	5
6	6
7	7

THE EIGHT ESSENTIALS OF LIFE

The Eight Essentials of the Healing Revolution are quite simple. These life-giving truths are not "new"; rather they have been largely lost and forgotten. It's time we excavate these jewels. Like deep secrets of the pyramids, we bring these ancient truths to light, using our healing tools to uncover and implement them.

Your choices in these eight simple domains can lead you to life, health, happiness and purpose. Popular health programs have suggested new diets, exercises, meditations or habits that will revolutionize your life. Some of these programs may be helpful. The Eight Essentials are unique in that they bring all health truths together into one whole. Get the Eight Essentials right and your life will truly be in balance.

A balance exists between all Eight Essentials. Each Essential affects the others. Each one interacts with the others. You are a whole person, therefore the approach to good health through the Eight Essentials is holistic and complete.

If you already feel overwhelmed, don't fret. A surprising fact about the Eight Essentials is that you don't have to work as hard as if you were focusing on one or a few of the areas of health. I've often seen stressed-out runners who torment their bodies so much that they sustain a permanent athletic injury. I've known many dieters who gave up because they couldn't lose any weight. These people have crashed and burned because they worked so hard in one essential area of life while neglecting the others.

> *The Eight Essentials enable you to work smarter, not harder. All eight systems support each other and work together in synergy, so that small positive steps in each area multiply for maximum combined results.*

The Eight Essentials enable you to work smarter, not harder. All eight systems support each other and work together in synergy, so that small, positive steps in each area multiply for maximum combined results. You can work smarter, not harder.

A lot of people are like a one-legged spider, barely dragging themselves along with one of these Eight Essentials. When they get two or three legs working, moving around becomes that much easier. Still, that spider is crippled and its world is small. When four or five legs are working, it might even get up on its feet. With six or seven legs moving in synch, that spider begins to dance. But with all eight legs in motion, life never looked so good. The other spiders start to take notice of that spider; it feels terrific and a universe of possibilities opens up to it. That's just what it's like to make positive changes with all of the Eight Essentials. I have seen many men and women literally start this journey like a one-legged spider, barely dragging themselves forward. I have seen many of them miraculously transformed into an eight-legged moving, grooving spider, simply by working smarter, not harder, with the Eight Essentials of life.

THE EIGHT ESSENTIALS ARE...

Life-destroying choices lead to:		Life-affirming choices lead to:
Depression, anxiety, apathy	1) The Human Spirit	Confidence, purpose, happiness
Overfed and undernourished	2) Nutrition	Health, appropriate weight
Stagnant fluids, dehydration	3) Water	Healthy, hydrated
Fatigue, weakness, obesity	4) Fitness	Strength, vigor, alertness
Perpetual tiredness	5) Sleep	Energy, well-rested, productivity
Stress, depression	6) Nature	Connected in nature
Alienation, unfulfillment	7) Relationships	Connected in community
Failure to thrive, early death	8) Hands On Techniques	Long life, generous givers
Human doers		**Human beings**

Any effort you make, however, is greatly impaired if you have negative attitudes and images of yourself. A positive attitude is *everything*. You won't go as far as you can when driven by a negative picture of what you do *NOT* want to be.

A POSITIVE ATTITUDE FOR HEALING

> *We know a great deal more about the causes of disease than we do about the causes of health.*
>
> *– Dr. M. Scott Peck*

Your *attitude* is your most important tool for activating health and wholeness. You are free to see yourself as healthy, happy and whole. Your attitude determines your altitude. You will become what you desire and believe about yourself.

Too many people have created sick, fat or unlovable images of themselves. They sabotage their healing by carrying these companions like apes around their necks. You cannot become on the outside what you are not on the inside. Once you shed the fat, sick or negative self-image, you will awaken to discover that the chains holding you back have been smashed. You will find the freedom to get up and run toward wholeness.

No human being is entitled to a negative attitude, even people with tragic handicaps or disabilities. Like a man in a wheelchair once said with a huge smile on his face, "I'm not crippled inside!" Or in the words of Nick Vujicic who was born with no arms or legs, "I won't pretend my life is easy, but through the love of my parents, loved ones, and faith in God, I have overcome my adversity and my life is now filled with joy and purpose."[14]

A happy life does not "happen to you." It is not dependent upon external circumstances. Joy is generated inside of you, despite external circumstances. Life grows from your heart.

Plant seeds of the charming, little old woman or man you hope to become, happily tending the garden of your life at 100 years of age, welcoming friends and family with a grin and a giggle (despite the disabilities you might have).

Desire.
Believe.
Become.

You are becoming outside what you desire and believe you can become inside. See yourself as whole, beautiful, strong and happy. Shed the negative images like reptile skins, never to pick them up again. A positive attitude is your most important tool.

CHOICE IS THE SPARK

Next, select one or more new life-affirming choices and take action. Don't wait until next week, tomorrow, or the end of this book to start your Healing Revolution. Do something today, no matter how small the first step might seem. Many people neglect to start because the journey seems daunting. This race is more for the plodding, persistent tortoise than it is for the sprinting hare.

Take a small step today. Make at least one positive, healthy choice related to your diet, drink, exercise, sleep, work, stress-management, relationships, daily routine or thoughts. Don't wait. Take that first step, then congratulate yourself for starting down the road to a more fulfilling life. If you are not sure what kind of changes to make, read on. The coming pages

---

14   *About Nick: His Story*, www.attitudeisaltitude.com/about-nick-his-story (January 2014).

have helpful, healthy suggestions to transform your life. Add more healthy choices to your daily routine as time goes by.

Begin by wholeheartedly implementing these changes for a month. See how you feel after a few weeks. See if you have more energy, if you are happier and if you are eager to embrace more positive changes. Implement the Healing Revolution and you will be hooked for life.

"Choice" is one of the key words of the Healing Revolution. Health is our birthright. It's a birthright that we _choose_ to receive. You and I are tempted _not_ to receive this birthright. We are tempted by all the unhealthy choices that come at us, nearly every step of the way in our journey from cradle to grave.

As for me, I choose to embrace the amazing birthright of life in all its abundance. If we listen to our instincts, we will discover that this amazing birth potential is hardwired within us. It is written in our genes. This birthright empowers us to make healthy choices, even if it has been dormant for most or all of our past years.

Choice is the spark that can awaken the blazing fire of life within us. Good choices revive and invigorate our passionate purpose in life, but bad choices can smother it. Choice has the power to liberate or enslave.

The power of choice is strong. We cannot enter into the age of the Healing Revolution without coming to grips with our choices. Making the right choices empowers each one of us to overcome mediocrity and live life with fullness and passion. Bad choices equal bad health. Good choices equal good health. Great choices equal great health.

As we press on further down this road into the Healing Revolution, I want to congratulate you for the choices you have made today. Make a bold entry in your journal. Tell your friends. Mark today's date in bright red on the calendar. This is a day to remember!

HAVE AN OPEN MIND

Have an open mind as I present some revolutionary tools designed to uncover deep truths that conventional methods cannot reveal, and which will provide strength to succeed where brute force and willpower fail. You might be uncertain or even skeptical of these more natural and intuitive tools and techniques. They might seem "new and strange" to you, but please know that they have been used to bring health and healing to many people for countless years.

Although modern researchers have amassed a huge library of data about conventional medicine, they are only beginning to understand the natural healing powers of the body, emotions, mind, prayer, meditation and Hands On Techniques (which are explained in the "HOT" chapter). The research results in these newer areas do, in fact, validate the importance of natural medicines and techniques. Moreover, many peoples' healing experiences confirm that the mind, spirit and Hands On Techniques are intricately linked to human well-being.

If you had lived long ago, your beloved friends and family might have thought you to be crazy if you set out to sail around the world. They would have feared for your life, lest you topple off the edge of the flat earth. Imagine the look of amazement on their faces when, after circumnavigating the globe, you sailed back safely into harbor.

Every generation is tempted to reject the things they cannot understand. Thankfully the days of flat earth medicine will soon be past – not that we reject all conventional medicine, but that we seek to enhance and refine it. We seek to free our powerful self-healing forces. So let us embrace these natural tools for tomorrow's better health, even if we do not fully understand them all.

I'm about to describe two powerful tools that we have developed and refined for nearly 40 years: the Muscle Response Test (MRT) and Tap Into Potential (TIP). These techniques will take you beyond the borders of flat earth medicine. Look to those who have already circumnavigated the globe using these tried and proven tools. Diverse theories exist about how these techniques work, but how they work is not so important as that *they do work*. I have personally seen many people use MRT and TIP for the improvement of their quality of life. Someday I will hopefully hear from you and learn how your life is better because of these safe and effective tools.

MUSCLE RESPONSE TEST (MRT)

The Muscle Response Test (MRT) is based on the concept that your body intuitively knows – more than your conscious mind – what therapies, substances, lifestyle choices or ideas are most beneficial for your health.[15]

15　MRT combines the best elements of other muscle testing modalities such as applied kinesiology, manual muscle testing and Nambudripad's Allergy Elimination Techniques (NAET).

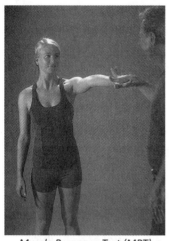

Muscle Response Test (MRT)

The basic theory is that your body exhibits a measurable muscle weakness when its bioenergetic field intersects with something dysfunctional or imbalanced.

According to one major review of more than 100 research studies, "manual muscle testing employed by chiropractors, physical therapists and neurologists was shown to be a clinically useful tool."[16] Articles published in medical journals have validated the reliability of muscle testing for dozens of different applications.[17] Still, all the research is useless for you if not put to the test. Give it a try right now!

You can use the Muscle Response Test to determine what lifestyle choices are good for your health. Combine MRT with Tap Into Potential (explained below) to identify and reprogram negative thought patterns. MRT can help you develop the positive attitudes and healthy lifestyles that are needed for your Healing Revolution in ways that conventional knowledge and testing cannot do. You have nothing to lose and everything to gain by trying MRT.

See Essential #8: Hands On Techniques, for specific instructions about how to use the Muscle Response Test (page 197). The coming chapters will show you how to use MRT specifically for each of the Eight Essentials. MRT gives you the power to discover and discern.

TAP INTO POTENTIAL (TIP)

Tap Into Potential (TIP) integrates a broad spectrum of safe and effective techniques that I have used with my patients.[18] The skeletal, muscular, immune, lymphatic, cardiovascular, urinary, digestive, respiratory, nervous, endocrine and reproductive systems are all enhanced by TIP. Tap Into Potential empowers people to accelerate their journey toward wholeness

---

16   Scott C. Cuthbert and George J. Goodheart, Jr., *On the Reliability and Validity of Manual Muscle Testing: A Literature Review,* Chiropractic & Osteopathy, 6 March 2007, 15(1):4.

17   *Research Supporting the Reliability of The Manual Muscle Test,* www.icakusa.com/files/Research-Reliability-of-the-Manual-Muscle-Test1.pdf (January 2014).

18   TIP is my way of integrating and enhancing the best elements of Applied Kinesiology, acupuncture, acupressure, Neuro Emotional Technique (NET), Nambudripad's Allergy Elimination Techniques (NAET), Emotional Freedom Technique (EFT) and Meridian Tapping.

and away from disease and self-limitation. TIP brings focus, clarity, confidence and strength.

You can use TIP to enhance the health of your skin, bones, joints, organs, mind, will and emotions. Use TIP to reprogram negative thought patterns and self-destructive attitudes. In the coming pages, I will tell you some amazing TIP success stories. I have known people, for example, who have overcome self-hate and addictions using TIP. I have known people who received relief from physical ailments and who reduced stress using TIP. I have helped patients eliminate fears of flying, fears of confrontation, fears of taking risks and fears of the unknown. Still TIP is not a magic cure-all. It is one very important part of a balanced, proactive, healthy, natural lifestyle.

TIP involves tapping your fingertips onto specific points on your body while making positive affirmations (vocally or in your thoughts) of health or healing. Tapping should be firm but not hard enough to cause pain.

Tap Into Potential is most effective

when done on special acupuncture meridian points. Meridians are neural pathways or energy channels in the body connecting a point on the skin with a specific organ. For centuries acupuncturists have directed their treatment toward points on the skin that are connected by meridians to the organs they wish to treat. TIP utilizes these same surface points and meridians. Dr. George Goodheart, the founder of Applied Kinesiology, recommended tapping in the temple region of the head to open up the body's filters and make it more receptive to healing. The other key tapping points I recommend include the top of your head (the "soft spot" when you were a baby), between your eyes, around both eyes, above and below the center of your lips, and on each side of your chest where your clavicle (collarbone) meets your sternum (breastbone).

TIP is perhaps most powerful when used in combination with the Muscle Response Test, with the help of a healing buddy. For example, have a friend use MRT to test your statement about a life-affirming change you desire to make.

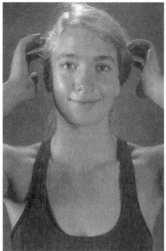

Tap Into Potential (TIP)

"I love exercise," you might say, or "I love fresh, green vegetables." Your friend may discover a MRT weakness when you make these statements, especially if you hate exercise or green vegetables. Then try tapping while repeating the statement "I love exercise" or "I love fresh, green vegetables." When your friend tests you again using MRT, you may discover new strength and resolve, especially after repeated application of the TIP techniques.

Use Tap Into Potential to correct sabotaging factors that have led to past failure in your life. I know of no other health procedure with as limitless a potential, with no negative side effects, with so many success stories and with absolutely no healthcare or insurance costs! You can experience positive results by simply investing five to 10 minutes each day in TIP and MRT. Many theories

👍 TRY THIS!

MRT and TIP for Great Health

(see Essential #8 to learn how to use MRT and TIP)

- *Begin by setting a target for your health. Set your target high. Even if you fall short, you will still be ahead.*
- *Use Muscle Response Test (MRT) to test statements such as, "I desire to be healed of_____. I desire to be healthy. I can be healthy. I will be healthy." Add your own words and goals.*
- *Use Tap Into Potential (TIP) to strengthen weak statements.*
- *Use MRT to re-test weak statements.*
- *Repeat until your healthy goals test strong and you see positive results in your life.*

WHO USES TAPPING?

Tapping is becoming more commonplace in hospitals and clinics, especially for dealing with pain and post-traumatic stress disorder. Some quotes from doctors: (EFT stands for Emotional Freedom Techniques, which is one form of tapping.)

"EFT offers great healing benefits."
– Deepak Chopra, MD

"Meridian-based therapies such as EFT...can have effects out of all proportion to their cost and complexity."
– Norm Shealy, MD, author of *Soul Medicine*

"EFT is at the forefront of the new healing movement."
– Candace Pert, PhD, author of *Molecules of Emotion*

"EFT is destined to be a top healing tool for the 21st century."
 – Cheryl Richardson, author of *The Unmistakable Touch of Grace*

"EFT is a simple, powerful process that can profoundly influence gene activity, health and behavior."
– Bruce Lipton, PhD, author of *The Biology of Belief*

"EFT is easy, effective, and produces amazing results. I think it should be taught in elementary school."
– Donna Eden, co-author of *The Promise of Energy Psychology*

"I frequently use EFT for my patients with great results."
– Eric Robins, MD, co-author of *Your Hands Can Heal You*

Other proponents of tapping include: Mehmet Oz, MD, Henry Altenberg, MD, Daniel J. Benor, MD, Irene A. Cohen, MD, Judith Friedman, MD, Gary Peterson, MD, Eric Robins, MD, Raul Vergini, MD, Joseph Mercola, DO, Cheryl Richardson, author, Christopher Hegarty, PhD, Nancy Steele, PhD, TSTA, Curtis Steele, MD, ABPN, Patricia Carrington, PhD, Inci Erkin, MD, Myron Koch, MD, David Lake, MD, Sandro de Rosa, MD, and Jack Canfield, co-author of *Chicken Soup for the Soul.*

exist as to why these tools work, but the important thing is that they do work. Those who reject what they do not understand will miss some rich rewards.

If you want to grow, tap. Don't wait for a healing buddy to test you. Don't wait to learn the "proper" technique. Tap in whatever way feels right to you and expect positive results. Tap each and every day. When in doubt, tap it out.

This has merely been a brief introduction to TIP. *For more specific instructions, see Essential 8: Hands On Techniques.*

IN CONCLUSION...

Our self-healing abilities are made to run on autopilot while keeping our minds, bodies and spirits in perfect health. The problem is, we've jammed the autopilot controls with a cluttered mess of stressful, unnatural influences. The temptation for busy people like you and me is to cram more fix-it programs into our schedule, which only adds to the stress. Instead of making a long "to-do list," we are learning to *become human beings* who naturally turn on the positive influences.

It's like the unruffled beagle who smiles in the face of the Doberman's threat, causing the Doberman to leave in search of a more fearful prey. Everybody respects confident, self-assured people who know who they are *becoming*. We don't have to *strive* if we believe in ourselves.

We are painting a positive, new picture of the healthy, happy people we are becoming. We are learning to be healthy human beings, not human doings. We are comfortable swaying with the natural rhythms of life, from sunshine to rain, rest to motion, fasting to eating, work to play and community to solitude. We rest in who we are and in our intrinsic self-worth, beauty and strength. We are putting our self-healing bodies back on autopilot.

We will look closer at these concepts and what it truly means to *be healthy humans* now, as we turn to Essential #1: Empowering the Human Spirit.

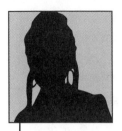

Renee's Story:
"My Problem is Ron"

Renee came into my practice with a problem that was difficult for her to verbalize. She was a fast-paced, type-A person, and she arrived with her husband Ron who was much more laid-back and mild. Renee's health assessment showed headaches and stress.

We treated Renee's stress and headaches with homeopathic remedies and chiropractic, although she was still bothered about something else. Gradually the primary reason for their visits rose to the surface.

"My problem is Ron," said Renee. "I don't love him. I don't even want him to touch me."

That's the sort of problem that most people don't take to a "regular" medical doctor. But in natural medicine, we treat the whole person. You can never assume that a relational problem, for example, isn't to blame for a physical ailment.

Renee and Ron had heard that our clinic was having success in out-of-the-ordinary cases, and they wanted to explore natural answers for their marital issues. I was able to quickly provide a homeopathic remedy to help Ron with a rather simple sexual problem. Then I focused on Renee.

"What is the main problem you are having with Ron," I asked.

"I'm just not attracted to him anymore."

"Has he been cheating on you?" I asked. "Or are you attracted to somebody else? Are you attracted to women? Do you have abuse issues in the past that are unresolved?"

Her answers were always in the negative. I was so perplexed. I saw no strong desire in her to reconcile with Ron, apart from the fact that she kept coming back to see me twice a week. Poor Ron was doing all that he could to make it work. They had three kids, so they also wanted to improve their marriage for the children's sake.

I tried Muscle Response Test with Renee.

I asked her to say "I love my husband."

"I love my husband," she said, and her arm went totally weak.

I could tell by the look on her face that this was not an easy statement for her to make. So I asked her to say, "I like my husband."

Her arm went weak with that one too.

"I want to fix things with my husband."

It was no good. She made it clear to me that she did not even want to say these words.

"How about this statement," I said. "I love my children."

Renee's arm was solid as a rock. Unfortunately I couldn't find anything she liked about her husband. She didn't even like driving in the car or eating dinner with him.

This was one of the toughest nuts I'd ever cracked. Why she didn't give up and go home, I'll never know. She was probably encouraged to continue coming to our clinic because we were able to help her with her stress and headaches.

At first she was opposed to our Tap Into Potential (TIP) techniques, but gradually she warmed up to the idea. I began by tapping in a circular pattern on her upper temple, and I taught her to tap there. This temporal sphenoidal area is helpful for bringing openness and receptivity to new ideas and attitudes.

Finally I found a chink in Renee's armor.

"Try saying this," I asked her. "I might like to possibly fix things with my husband."

"I might like to possibly fix things with my husband," she repeated while I tapped her TIP points.

The Muscle Response Test showed her arm to be strong!

Now we're getting somewhere, I thought.

"Now say this: I might want to love my husband."

She went weak. We began to tap the TIP points, and then I continued more gradually.

"I might like our friendship to improve a little."

Her arm was strong.

Like a goat climbing a craggy cliff, we found a twisting path through affirmative statements that she was willing to say about her husband.

"Ron has good intentions," she would say while tapping. "He has good qualities. He is a good father and a good friend to his friends. I remember being attracted to Ron when we first met."

Her homework assignment was to tap the active acupuncture points that tested positive, while making statements of affirmation about Ron. Within a week, Renee was saying with confidence, "I want to like my husband. I want to love my husband. I want our marriage to get better." Her muscle tested strong when she made these statements.

Still I perceived a slight grimace on her face when she talked about Ron. I took her only as far and as fast as she wanted to go. Within three weeks, her husband Ron pulled me aside.

"I don't know what you're doing," he said, "but keep it up. It's working. She's a lot more fun to be around." He gave me a wink, and I knew the spring thaw was underway.

Renee herself didn't yet believe she had made any significant change of attitude, even though muscle testing showed that she was making good progress. She was still a skeptic.

"I'm probably wasting my money," she told me.

"No you're not," I urged. "Just stick with this a few more sessions, okay?"

Within about a month she was saying "I love Ron" with strong, positive results and with no frown. We addressed other issues from the Eight Essentials that she and Ron could improve upon. When I'd taken these love birds as far as I could, I cut the strings and let them go. And fly they did.

When the report card came out at their next quarterly visit, Renee got straight As. She and Ron were happily married. They enjoyed eating together, laughing together and going on dates together. Ron confided in me that their physical intimacy which had really suffered before was now off the charts.

That just goes to show you how far you can go, even if you only might want to possibly someday (maybe) think about committing to the Healing Revolution – no promises.

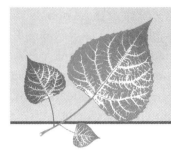

ESSENTIAL #1: EMPOWERING THE HUMAN SPIRIT

Whether you think you can or you can't, you're right. – **Henry Ford**

Here's an incredible story that was reported widely in the media: Doctors told Sam Shoeman of Nashville, Tennessee, that he had just a few months to live. Medical scans showed extensive cancerous growths on his left liver lobe.

Sam Shoeman was devastated. He only wanted one thing: to survive three months until Christmas. If he could spend the holidays at home with the ones he loved, his life would be complete.

Sam Shoeman had a meaningful Christmastime with his family. Then he was readmitted to the hospital on New Year's Day. Within 24 hours, Sam Shoeman was dead.

There's nothing strange about this true story ... except that Sam Shoeman never had terminal cancer.

That's right. He had no physical reason to die.

Sam Shoeman *thought* he had terminal cancer because of his liver scan, but ... it turns out that his liver scan was botched. The autopsy revealed a tiny spot of cancerous tissue that could not have possibly killed Sam Shoeman.

So what killed Sam Shoeman?

Doctors determined that he died of psychosomatic causes. His mind told his body when he was supposed to die, and his body obeyed, right on cue.[19]

Similarly, researchers have documented "voodoo deaths," such as that of a Maori tribal woman who ate a piece of fruit and an African man who ate a wild hen. Both died within 24 hours of learning that the harmless food they ate was cursed with a killing taboo.

---

19   Nigel Barber, *Voodoo Death I*, www.psychologytoday.com/blog/the-human-beast/201209/voodoo-death-i (January 2014).

Like Sam Shoeman, both of these people's sense of panic and helplessness was reinforced by the absolute conviction of friends and relatives that the victim was doomed and would surely die. Like Sam Shoeman, their hearts stopped beating because their expectations became a self-fulfilling prophecy.

MIND OVER MATTER

The body is bioenergetic as well as biochemical. You are more than a corpse, because a corpse is just chemicals. Medical science doesn't have the instruments and technology to comprehend the body's bioenergetic control forces – not yet – but don't let that fact close your mind to the mysteries of the mind and spirit. Only flat earth proponents reject the things they do not understand. Voodoo death and the placebo effect are just two manifestations of how this bioenergetic force interacts with the tangible health of mind, body, will and emotions.

Like yin and yang, voodoo death is the dark side of a force that can also be used for good. The placebo effect is one expression of that powerful force. Patients in double-blind trials who believed they were receiving an effective drug or surgery – but who in fact received fake treatment – actually had ulcers healed, blood pressure reduced, bronchi dilated and warts reduced. Bald men who believed they were receiving legitimate treatment – but were not – actually grew hair. [20]

Similarly, a large number of patients who were told they might experience negative side effects of a drug or treatment – but who in fact received fake medication – experienced the same symptoms they were warned of, which included fatigue, vomiting, headaches, memory loss and more. Worse yet, surgery patients who were "convinced" of their impending death usually died during surgery, while patients who were merely "unusually apprehensive" about death, survived.

Science has only begun to scratch the surface of comprehension into the self-healing and self-killing power and potential of the human will. Epigenetics, as discussed in the previous chapter, is coming to understand

---

20   Lissa Rankin, *The Nocebo Effect: How Negative Thoughts Can Harm Your Health*, www.positivelypositive.com/2013/01/23/the-nocebo-effect-how-negative-thoughts-can-harm-your-health/ (January 2014).

the astonishing human ability to rise above genetic "destiny" and determine a new, life-giving course for the future. You literally hold the power to shape your future. The question is, what will you do with this power?

Perhaps it depends upon your self-image and how you see yourself.

VICTIM OR VICTOR?

You are the Director of your own Health Department.
You can end your own Healthcare Crisis.
You are your own Supreme Court, handing down your life or death sentence.
You are the Hero of your own epic drama.
You choose your main character – either Victim or Victor.
You are your Doctor, with chart and pen in hand, ready to write your own prescription.
Therefore, the question is ...
What do you want to be?... a Victim or a Victor?

Unfortunately, _you_ just might be the biggest obstacle to your healing. Do not sabotage your healing. Don't be tempted to shift the blame for your health on others, when the power to heal is within you. You cannot blame your ancestors, chromosomes, social class, schooling, employment status, financial status, chronic illnesses, habits, climate, family, friends or even the bad things that have happened to you. The choice is yours.

Voices all around tempt us to believe that the pleasurable, unnatural, unhealthy choices of the modern world – which lead to chronic sickness and early death – are better than a long, healthy, happy life. Hospitals are filled with people who are sick and dying young because they said "yes" to all of the deceptive choices that the commercial world has given them. Many of these poor people will never know what killed them. But now you know better, so choose life!

Believe in your healing. Believe in who you are becoming. You and the world around you will be a better place when you are at the top of your

> *Anyone who stops learning is old, whether at twenty or eighty. Anyone who keeps learning stays young. The greatest thing in life is to keep your mind young.*
>
> *– Henry Ford*

game. I wish I could find the words to tell you how valuable you are, how much your life matters, how you are one-of-a-kind, and how much the world needs you to be healthy and whole, bringing your talents and joy to the people around you.

You are a beautiful, wonderfully-crafted person, a one-of-a-kind masterpiece. Don't sabotage your healing. You are receiving the knowledge and power to grasp hold of the abundant life. I can't do it for you. Your doctor can't do it for you. A social worker can't do it for you. Only you can do it for you!

Choose a long, healthy and abundant life!

EMPOWER YOURSELF

> *Be sober and temperate, and you will be healthy. Be in general virtuous, and you will be happy.*
>
> *– Benjamin Franklin*

Country music totally transformed my life ... but only when I started listening to the songs backwards. That's when my wife came home, my pa got out of jail, the truck got fixed, the bank gave me back my farm and my lost dog got found.[21]

The world is full of sad, "somebody done somebody wrong songs." Tax men, bosses, advertisers, in-laws and outlaws want to "do" your life their way, not yours. The question is, what story do you want to be written for your life? Only you can dis-empower others by cutting the strings of control they have on your life, your health, your attitudes and your emotions. Only *you* can empower yourself. You are accountable for your health and wholeness, not the tax man, not your friends, not your family, not your boss, not the government, not even your doctor.

You are in charge of your personal joy meter, and only you can turn it up or turn it down. I think of my mother who was the most cheerful old lady you'd ever meet up until the day she died, even though she had the same aches and pains as many other people her age. I remember 80-year-old Paul Bragg who amazed us young people by lecturing on his head, and yet we never heard him say one word of complaint about anything. You

---

21   For more on the topic, see Rascal Flatt's song "Backwards" off their 2006 album "Me and My Gang."

might know a spry old codger who fits that description. That's the kind of person you can become, despite your circumstances. You are writing your own life story. What kind of a main character do you choose to become: a victim? … or a victor?

Bad or unpleasant things may happen to you, but those things cannot take your joy, your peace or your happiness. Only you can give those priceless gems away. Turn up the joy meter. Be a victor, not a victim. You will be healthier and more whole if you look for good even in difficult situations. You are the gardener. What creative life are you cultivating in the garden of your heart?

Let us get rid of one misconception: Doctors do not "heal." Your body heals itself. All doctors can do is help (or hinder) that healing. In nearly four decades of practice, the best treatment I have ever given my patients is to empower them to accept that they are in charge of their own healing.

> *Each morning when I open my eyes I say to myself: I, not events, have the power to make me happy or unhappy today. I can choose which it shall be. Yesterday is dead, tomorrow hasn't arrived yet. I have just one day, today, and I'm going to be happy in it.*
>
> *— Actor*
> **Groucho Marx**

- ◆ *Only you can control your choices and your lifestyle.*
- ◆ *You are your best doctor, on call 24 hours a day, seven days a week.*
- ◆ *Ask not what your doctor can do for you, but what you can do for you.*
- ◆ *The healthcare crisis starts and ends with you (and each one of us).*
- ◆ *No disease on this planet is too strong for your healthy body to cure.*

Empower your human spirit by cutting the chains that bind you and by saying, "YES! I accept life, joy, happiness and health exceedingly, abundantly more than I have yet imagined."

Flat earth medicine is satisfied when it eliminates symptoms. As long as the patient is still breathing, flat earth medicine has done its job. But flat earth medicine can never awaken the healing power within you.

Are you satisfied with flat earth medicine? I'm not! I'm breaking out of flat earth thinking by way of the Healing Revolution!

The amazing person you hope to become starts within you. It permeates your spirit, mind, heart, will, emotions and body. Accept the fact that your life and health can improve exceedingly, abundantly more than you have yet imagined.

Realize the truth that you are designed to be healthy. Great health, happiness and a fulfilling life are within your grasp.

KEYS TO HAPPINESS

These are some simple day-to-day habits that will help increase happiness in your life.

◆ *Savor everyday moments. I love tuning into the simple things that bring joy to life each day. Stop to smell the roses and find beauty in people and the amazing life all around you.*

◆ *Create! We, more than any other creatures on earth, are born to create. This creative energy is at the heart of the Healing Revolution. You might not be a painter or musician, but you can create something of beauty to share with others. Creating is one of your most profound keys to happiness.*

◆ *Avoid comparisons. Comparisons cripple your self-worth and lead you to make bad decisions.*

◆ *Live more simply and don't stress about money. Worry leads to depression and anxiety.*

◆ *Eat simple, natural foods and drink pure, natural spring water. Bad diets lead to depression.*

◆ *Cultivate goals and purpose. Significant dreams and aspirations lead to deeper joy and purpose.*

◆ *Find passion in your work. The wrong work attitude can suck the life out of you.*

◆ *Invest in friends and family. Develop at least a few long-lasting, caring, healthy relationships.*

◆ *Resolve conflict and practice forgiveness, even if you do not receive kindness in return.*

◆ *Smile and have a positive attitude. Even if you don't feel like it, an optimistic attitude goes a long way in lifting spirits.*

◆ *Exercise outdoors. Fresh air, sunshine and exercise work wonders on both the mind and body.*

◆ *Tune into your healthy intuitions, which will lead you to make positive, life-affirming choices in all Eight Essentials of life.*

◆ *Give generously. The health benefits of giving time and money are higher than quitting smoking. Your feelings about yourself improve dramatically when you help others in need.*

TRY THIS! FUTURES DIARY

Paint a picture of who you are becoming by writing a Futures Journal (which might be one part of your more-inclusive Health Journal). This is a to-be list rather than a to-do list. Describe what you hope your life will look like in a month, a year or in ten years. Note your best qualities, for example: "I will be fun and sassy, always with a smile, a song, a joke or a word of encouragement for others. I'll have plenty of time to help others. I'll buy whole foods from the farmer's markets and roadside stands. My sore joints will be stronger."

Be as specific as you like with physical, mental, emotional and spiritual attributes. Tap your way to success with TIP. Keep this picture of who you are becoming always in your mind. Regularly add new entries about who you hope to become.

I remember the time I was parking my car in a public lot and – on a whim – I gave the parking attendant five extra bucks.

"That's for the car behind me," I said.

"Right," said the attendant, not knowing that I didn't have a clue who was in the car behind me.

I was walking away from my parked car when a guy came running.

"Hey!" he shouted. "Did you just pay for my parking?"

"Yeah," I said. I watched his jaw drop in astonishment.

"Wow," he said. "That was amazing. Thank you so much!"

You would have thought he had won the lottery by the look on his face. Of course my smile was no less radiant. That's how one simple gesture can kick somebody's joy level up through the goal posts.

The centurions who live in the world's "Blue Zones" intuitively know many of the keys to happiness. These people all have regular stress-relieving moments built into their daily routine; times when they pause to remember ancestors, pray, nap or meet with friends for wine and dance. Most of them draw a sense of purpose from faith-based communities. As a rule they live in close connection with their family and friends. They regularly exercise their minds and bodies.[22]

A survey of 14,000 men and women determined that people are happier if they:

◆ *Watch TV or play video games less than 30 minutes each day.*
◆ *Spend no more than one hour on social networks per day.*
◆ *Listen to more than an hour of music every day.*
◆ *Spend time volunteering each week.*
◆ *Have at least one friend of a different race or ethnicity.*
◆ *Get 8 to 9 hours of sleep per night.*
◆ *Practice relaxation techniques like yoga or meditation.*
◆ *Take more vacation days each year.*
◆ *Get more sunshine and spend time in nature every day.*
◆ *Read at least 6 books each year.* [23]

TRY THIS!   MRT AND TIP: SELF IMAGE

(see Essential #8 to learn how to use MRT and TIP)

• *It's difficult to move forward as long as you are tied to the image of who you once were. You are not the sick, fat, fatigued or undisciplined person you used to be. Leave those images behind.*

• *Use Muscle Response Test (MRT) and Tap Into Potential (TIP) to reprogram a negative self-image.*

• *Tap statements describing who you are becoming, such as, "I am a new person. Even if I still look the same on the outside, I am different inside. I am becoming a beautiful, new person. I am at peace with myself. I am focusing on my strengths, which are _____ ."*

• *Use MRT to test your progress on these same statements.*

Moreover, imagine how much happier these 14,000 people would be if their daily habits covered all Eight Essentials, including good nutrition, water

---

22   According to Dan Buettner (*Blue Zones*), family interaction lowers disease and mortality rates for both elderly people and the children in the home, and committing to a life partner adds up to three years of life expectancy.

23   Dan Buettner, *Thrive* (Washington, DC: National Geographic Society, 2011), p. 251-259.

and fitness. This kind of thoughtful, holistic, healthy lifestyle leads to joy that is fuller and less transient than a superficial happiness that comes and goes. What's more, people with a deep-seated, unwavering joy can expect to add an extra decade to their lives.[24]

How is your joy meter? You can find ways to crank up the joy by taking a free Whole Person Appraisal at www.DrFrankKing.com. The more joy you cultivate, the fuller your reservoir will remain. Keep your joy full by practicing the Eight Essentials on a daily basis. Keep filling your reservoir until you have an ocean of joy that is not swayed by the storms of life.

ATTITUDES AND EMOTIONS

A cheerful heart is good medicine. –

King Solomon

– (Proverbs 17:22)

Do you lack joy or feel depressed? Fight depression by bringing joy to others. Do you feel unloved and unfriended? Your best remedy is to act in love and be a friend to others. Are you angry or anxious? Your best remedy is to generate peace. Whatever negative attitudes and emotions trouble you, seek ways to generate the opposite, healthy attitudes and emotions.

Research has shown that positive attitudes and emotions improve mental health, longevity, cardio-vascular health and recovery from surgery. People who handle stress better have lower levels of inflammation and a stronger immune system. Positive attitudes dramatically improve healing. "When a person can focus on something other than illness, it allows the body to take advantage of our own healing capacity," says Dr. Herbert Benson of Harvard Medical School.[25]

On the other hand, people who cultivate a fear of anything from car accidents to cancer make themselves more vulnerable to the very thing they fear. A positive, confident attitude will get you and keep you out of trouble.

My experience in natural health and private practice has convinced me that every attitude and emotion has a direct impact on health, for good or for bad. I have seen how resentment and bitterness are related to gallbladder and liver illnesses. Fear seems to be related to kidney

---

24   Ibid, p. 244.
25   Sharon Jayson, *Power of a Super Attitude*, usatoday30.usatoday.com/news/health/2004-10-12-mind-body_x.htm (January 2014).

dysfunctions. Internalized anger and stress seem to contribute to problems of arthritis. Internalized shame, guilt, apathy, grief, anxiety, stress and hate are all like poison to the body.[26]

Thankfully you can strengthen your health by replacing negative attitudes with positive ones like acceptance, thankfulness, forgiveness, trust, optimism, willingness, understanding, love, joy, faith, peace and serenity. Find a healing buddy – a friend or family member – to help you identify negative issues that you will want to remove and replace. For difficult cases, visit a natural-focused professional. Never dwell too much on the negative. If you were in a dark, muddy pit with your hands on a rope, you may be tempted to stare at your mucky feet. Instead, salvation is found by looking up toward the light, grabbing the rope and pulling yourself up. Imagine the sunshine and breezes. Picture the new you that you want to become. Then simply rise up and *become the new you!*

> *When you are inspired by some great purpose, some extraordinary project, all your thoughts break their bonds: Your mind transcends limitations, your consciousness expands in every direction, and you find yourself in a new, great, and wonderful world. Dormant forces, faculties and talents become alive, and you discover yourself to be a greater person by far than you ever dreamed yourself to be.*
>
> *– Hindu guru and yoga master Patanjali*

Desire.
Believe.
Become.

Your attitude determines your altitude, so fly high and far. Take back the control of your attitudes and emotions. Muscle Response Test (MRT), Tap Into Potential (TIP) and my Whole Person Appraisal at www.DrFrankKing. com are three effective tools to help renew and revitalize your attitudes and emotions.

---

26   Ken Cohen, *The Way of Qigong : The Art and Science of Chinese Energy Healing* (New York: Random House, 1997).

IT TAKES AN ARMY FOR A REVOLUTION

Good habits are contagious, but so are bad habits. Your community is one of the most important factors influencing the outcome of the Healing Revolution in your life.

Let's be honest: You might have the best health intentions in the world, but if the advertisers of commercialism continually bombard you with messages undermining your health, if your family members pack your kitchen shelves with junk food, and if your friends cram your mind with junk attitudes, you are fighting a steep, uphill battle.

You will want partners on this positive path to life. It's a primal, tribal part of who we are. If your tribe is swirling down into the garbage dump, you will likely be dragged down with them. But if you have a climbing partner to help belay you out of the dark pit of death, away from the zombie life forms, up onto the mountains where healing streams gurgle through flower-studded meadows, then you will succeed.

Do not underestimate the destructive power of constant, negative messages from your friends, family and the media. Personally connect with people and groups who share your yearning for abundant life.

For example, Pastor Rick Warren made a significant observation about his Saddleback Church in Southern California.

"We have a big church," he said.

And he wasn't referring to numbers. He meant body fat, a conspicuous sin of the flesh that plagued Rick Warren and his followers.

Rick Warren joined with three doctors to form a weight loss program called the Daniel Plan. Accountability to other people is a centerpiece of the Daniel Plan. In the first year, 15,000 participants collectively lost 250,000 pounds. People who participated in support groups lost twice as much weight as those who followed the program alone. Rick Warren himself lost 60 pounds.[27]

It takes an army of like-minded people to initiate a revolution.

---

27 *The Daniel Plan*, www.DanielPlan.com and Nanci Hellmich, *Pastor Rick Warren Born Again to Healthier Living*, yourlife. usatoday.com/fitness-food/diet-nutrition/story/2012-02-05/Pastor-Rick-Warren-born-again-to-healthier-living/52975790/1 (January 2014).

FAITH AND PURPOSE

Paint a picture in your mind of the YOU that you hope to become.
Imagine that ...

◆ *your body is healthy,*
◆ *your mind is happy,*
◆ *your smile is bright,*
◆ *you have a terrific attitude,*
◆ *you have abundant energy,*
◆ *you have discovered your life mission and purpose, and*
◆ *your joy is infectious to people around you.*

TRY THIS!   TIP: FACE YOUR FEARS

(see page 201 for help using TIP)

- *Use Tap Into Potential (TIP) to eliminate fear.*
- *Rate your fear on a scale of 0 to 10, with 0 being "no fear" and 10 being "maximum fear."*
- *Use TIP while affirming that you are not afraid. Be creative, stating in different ways that fear has no power over you, that it is gone, that it doesn't affect you, that it is replaced with peace.*
- *After a few minutes of tapping, rate your fear again.*
- *Repeat the procedure and keep rating your fear. Most people find that their fear level decreases substantially.*
- *The next time you face the object of your fear, find your place of peace and enjoy your new freedom!*

This is a picture of the new you. This image of health will lead you deeper into the Healing Revolution. Faith and persistence will help you to resist all the destructive choices. Your positive image of health will lead you on the ascending path to wholeness.

Many people look to a "higher power" to succeed. The Alcoholics Anonymous support group, for example, profess, "[We] believe that a Power greater than ourselves could restore us to sanity."[28] Faith in a higher power

---

28   Alcoholics Anonymous, *Twelve Steps and Twelve Traditions* (New York: Alcoholics Anonymous World Services, Inc., 2004).

gives people strength and a sense of purpose amid popular messages that undermine self-worth. Research shows that faith contributes to longevity, and that attending faith-based services four times per month add four to 14 years of life expectancy.[29]

I attribute healing energy to a Higher Power. I have seen this power confirmed through miraculous events in my life and in my patient's lives for nearly 40 years. In simplest terms, this is what I call "God." Taoists point to a power called chi. Homeopathy's founder Samuel Hahnemann attributed healing to what he called the "life force." You may use whatever words suit you best, or use no words at all.

Ask for help – I do that every day. I could not have received such abundant blessings for myself and my patients if I had not asked for help, answers, insights and solutions. Faith and a sense of purpose help us reap the benefits of greater health and happiness. You, too, can benefit from an attitude of faith and expectation. Ask for help in every aspect of your life. Seek revelation for your life purposes.

If you want to grow into something better, paint a clear picture of the person that you hope to become. Hold that vision of health and happiness close to your heart. You are created for wholeness and don't let anybody tell you otherwise. You are a unique and important asset to the human community. Without your creative strength and beauty, the world would be a poorer place.

Continually paint that picture of a strong, handsome, witty and creative *you* in your mind. Keep that picture always before you. Make that picture an attitude that sustains you in the Healing Revolution. Continue to refine your vision. Ask your Higher Power for help in refining you and taking you beyond your own abilities.

Never forget who you are becoming.

HUMAN DOINGS

Often the human response to a message like this is a feeling of exhaustion and defeat at the overwhelming list of personal improvements to be made. You might be tempted to work really, really hard to "fix all the screwed up things in your life." Or more likely, you will get depressed and give up.

---

29   Donna Fuscaldo, *How to Live to 100...and Beyond*, www.foxbusiness.com/personal-finance/2012/07/31/how-to-live-to-100and-beyond/ (January 2014).

Here is the key: Know that you are not a "human doing" but a "human being." Empowering the human spirit does not mean *doing* more but rather *being* more. It means securing that healthy, complete picture of yourself as an awesome human being, regardless of circumstances, regardless of other people's expectations.

Use Tap Into Potential (TIP; page 201) to reprogram your self-image, to help you see yourself as a healthy, successful, whole and fulfilled person. This is your destiny. This is your genetic potential. This is your joy, to become a whole human BE-ing.

Think of the underdog athlete who surprises everybody by coming from behind, or the sickly child who survives and grows to astound the world with innovative contributions for humanity. Think of the poor "nobody" who rises from the ashes to revolutionize history. These people are simply being who they were born to be. They saw the picture of their potential. Then they lived the picture.

Live your picture. Become a whole human "BE-ing."

DESIRE, BELIEVE, BECOME

You have painted a picture of the *you* that you want to become. Or maybe you have simply painted a picture of one small part of the new you.

With that picture in your mind, these are the three magic words of the Healing Revolution. You have already seen them in the previous pages, and you will see them again:

Desire.
Believe.
Become.

*Say what you **desire**: "I want to be healthy."* Desire is the will to be well. It is the catalyst for change. It is the first step as you drill down toward your center. Use Tap Into Potential (TIP) to reinforce your new, life-affirming desires.

*Say what you **believe**: "I believe I can be healthy."* Your belief takes you closer to your core, closer to authenticity. You are halfway along the journey from human doing to human being. Again, use TIP to help reprogram your beliefs.

> *Man often becomes what he believes himself to be. If I keep on saying to myself that I cannot do a certain thing, it is possible that I may end by really becoming incapable of doing it. On the contrary, if I have the belief that I can do it, I shall surely acquire the capacity to do it even if I may not have it at the beginning.*
>
> *– Mahatma Gandhi*

Say what you are **becoming**: "I am healthy." Now you reach the bedrock, the core of your being. Your picture is real. Your mind, body, attitudes and emotions are freed to truly be the human you were meant to be. Negative circumstances cannot touch your emotions and attitudes anymore.

To break free from your gray past and rise into the blue skies of your abundant future, reinforce these attitudes with TIP. We may not know exactly how it works; we only know that tapping does work ... in a profoundly, powerful way. I have counseled many people on this journey that you are now taking, and my greatest joy is to watch them walk into the victorious, abundant life that awaits them.

You might say, "I **desire** to break free from *[fill in the blank]* that imprisons me."

Then start living as if you are free.

"I **believe** I can break these chains," you say.

Then paint a picture of the new, liberated you, using TIP to empower you.

"I am a victor," you say, "not a victim." Grasp hold of that new vision and become it. Without vision, the people perish.

*Whatever your need is, fill it on the inside and you
will become it on the outside.
Don't think problems. Think solutions. Think wholeness.
Receive a new, victorious image of who you are becoming.
Empower your human spirit with this image of wholeness.
Awaken the new, victorious life and healing power within you.
Embrace wholeness throughout your entire mind, will, emotions, choices,
beliefs and self-image.
Believe until you become.
This is the creative power of the human spirit in action.*

SELF-EVALUATION
EMPOWERING the HUMAN SPIRIT

My Life-Destroying Choices
(e.g.: low self-image, negative attitudes, isolation, feeling like a victim)

My Life-Affirming Choices
(e.g.: believe in myself, accept challenges and victories, know I am beautiful, value life and health)

My Life-Destroying Choices	My Life-Affirming Choices
1	1
2	2
3	3
4	4
5	5
6	6
7	7

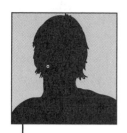

Roger's Story:
Seeing the Light

"Roger. Roger?"

He just sat there in my office, glazed eyes staring at the wall.

"Come on, Roger."

I gently shook him. He was slow to respond, as if heavily sedated.

"Hey Roger. Give me your attention, okay?"

Gradually he recovered, gaining focus.

Roger was a psychologist and he was very depressed. He was a deep thinker and he had a habit of internalizing other people's problems. His private practice was going downhill because he was so depressed that he could hardly function anymore.

"I just can't shake these feelings," he told me.

The roots of depression were easy to trace, leading straight to his counseling sessions. As Roger counseled his patients, he heard their problems, he analyzed their problems, he took on their problems, he became obsessed with their problems, and eventually he *became* their problems.

I've seen this same problem with other people, like the mother who is so intent upon removing her child's pain that she begins to physically feel her child's pain. This actually happened to me once in my practice. I had been treating so many sciatic nerve cases that I became consumed with the pathology of the problem, rather than the solution. Motivated by empathy, I began to feel the pain in my own sciatic nerve. I even walked with a limp until I recognized the problem and learned to manage my thoughts and emotions.

I explained to Roger that as a compassionate healer, he needed to step back and practice empathy from an appropriate distance. It wasn't his job to carry their pain, but only to help relieve their pain.

I suggested that Roger make some statements of positive affirmation that would take his attitudes in a healthy direction.

"I don't need to focus on my patients' problems. I will not focus on their pain. I will not take their pain. I cannot take their problems."

Roger repeated these statements while tapping key acupuncture points on his head.

"I don't need to analyze all aspects of the problem. I will not remain in the problem. I release the problem. I will focus on the solution. From now on, I am focusing on the solution. I will help people live in the solution."

As in most cases, many different aspects of the Eight Essentials contributed to his depression. Roger spent most of the day sitting at his desk in an office building. He had a poor diet and was gaining weight. He watched a lot of TV at night and had trouble sleeping.

Over the next two weeks, Roger made slow but steady progress. He made positive changes in all of the Eight Essentials. He ate better, exercised more, enjoyed nature and drank more water. His whole attitude toward life steadily improved.

I remember the afternoon Roger lit up like a Roman candle. He finally "got it." The session began in darkness when I turned off the lights.

"The darkness is your problem," I said. "You are surrounded by problems, Roger. What eliminates problems? More darkness? What can eliminate the darkness?"

"Light," said Roger.

I turned on a flashlight.

"The light is the solution, Roger. You cannot fight darkness with darkness, but only with light. So what do you want to focus on? The darkness or the light?"

He didn't hesitate. "I want to focus on the light."

We turned on the overhead light and he began tapping while repeating statements of positive affirmation.

"I will focus on the solutions," I said.

"I will focus on the solutions," he said.

"No more darkness for me. I will focus on the light." He kept repeating the affirmations that I made while he tapped.

"The light is so strong that it eliminates the darkness. The darkness is gone. All I can see now is the light."

That's when something clicked. That's when the fireworks went off and Roger finally "got it."

"The problems don't mean anything anymore," Roger said without my prompting. "It's all about the solutions now. It all about the light. The light is powerful. The light is overwhelming. The light is consuming me!"

My jaw dropped as I sat back and watched Roger move into high gear. His voice raised in volume and intensity.

"It's the light that destroys darkness. It's the light that heals me. It's the light that gives me life. It's the light that gives me energy."

His eyes and smile were so bright, he didn't look like the same man anymore. He could hardly get the words out fast enough.

"It's the light that will transform my patients. It's the light that provides solutions. It's the light that brings freedom. It's the light that not only smashes the problems, but brings solid, life-changing answers. The darkness is nothing! These problems are nothing! The light is everything!"

He shouted the words with authority. A wave of healing power overwhelmed Roger. I physically *felt* that power fill the room, same as the light that had filled every crack of darkness.

That was Roger's big breakthrough. And it wasn't just a momentary high; he was truly transformed from that point onward.

I love watching the light go on in people's lives. I've seen this same story happen over and over again ... same story, different characters. This flash of light is the epiphany moment that makes a professional doctor's job superfluous. For me, it's like delivering a new baby, born again into the Healing Revolution.

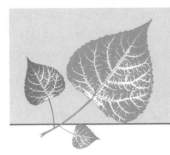

ESSENTIAL #2:
NUTRITION

You should eat to live,

not live to eat.

— Socrates

My mother was the Cool Whip Queen – she'd smother her famous pies and angel food cake with heaps of the luscious stuff. Her warm berry cobbler with fresh vanilla ice cream and strawberry shortcake was the best. My brothers and I believed it was food for the gods.

I was raised on the farm, where hard work is fueled by mountains of good grub. We didn't know anything about health food back then. We were standard meat-and-potatoes Midwesterners, with plenty of our own beef and sweet corn. Sometimes we'd even pick dandelion greens from the lawn and my mother would boil them for dinner.

I loved gathering berries with the neighbor kids. If we didn't have a basket to put the berries in, we'd thread the plump blackberries down the long, thin stalks of timothy grass like buttons on a string, 20 berries or more to a stem. We'd have a contest to see who could gather the most fruit, but I only cared about stuffing my belling with ripe berries right off the vine. Still, I always brought some home, since berries in the freezer meant more pies and cobblers from the Cool Whip Queen.

My first health food lesson came from my dad, who wouldn't allow soft drinks in the house. "That stuff will rust your pipes," he would say. We didn't know any more about nutrition than the average family back then.

Then an odd duck named Karl came into my life. He rented a small house from my dad along the main highway. Karl wore scruffy clothes and had hair growing everywhere, from his bushy head to his thick mono-brow. It sprouted from his ears and actually grew across the top of his nose. His Neanderthal-like appearance was intensified when he spoke to me in his thick, Eastern-European accent.

"Hello, Frankie," he'd say, his bright eyes sparkling beneath the overhanging brows. "How are you today, Frankie?"

His sweet, little wife was a white-haired babushka, every bit as strange and wonderful as Karl.

I liked going for walks with Karl.

"Hey Frankie," he'd say, touching a sapling. "D'you know what this is? It's sassafras, Frankie. You can tell by the three-lobed leaves. Peel back the bark like this, Frankie, and you can chew on it. It tastes good. You can also eat the roots."

He taught me how to make sassafras tea from the roots. He showed me licorice and other edible plants that grow in the wild. He let me read his Organic Gardening Magazines. He gave me some amazing produce from a large vegetable and herb garden behind his house. Karl had a magical touch in the garden, but as far as I'm concerned, the greatest seed he ever planted was the love of nature in my heart.

THE FAMILY FARM

I was a late-comer to my father, who was 49 years old when I was born. So when I was in my teens and my dad went into part-time retirement, my older brothers took charge of the country restaurant and motel, leaving me primarily in charge of the family farm. This was at a time when I was becoming very excited about nutrition and healthy living. I learned how far we had digressed from the natural roots of agriculture. That's when I drew a line in the dirt, metaphorically speaking, and said, "The food from our land will be natural, healthy, whole and free of chemicals." So in the early 1970s, I converted our 450 acres to a more healthy farm, using organic and biodynamic principles.

Americans will eat garbage, provided you sprinkle it liberally with ketchup.

— Author Henry James

Once upon a time, natural farms and gardens fed us. We caught and raised natural fish and meats. Then farming corporations arrived, applying what was learned in the Industrial Revolution to mass-food production. Trucks and trains carried the food to factories, not local markets. These factories did their wonder-working magic on the food, processing it, enhancing the taste with artificial flavors, adding artificial nutrients, increasing its shelf life, and of course, multiplying profits for corporations.

I can't help but wonder how chemical concoctions like diet sodas or breakfast cereals with 55 percent sugar ever got to be classified as "food."

While we were not paying attention, factories – not farms – put their products on the shelves of our markets. While our heads were turned, factories – not farms – placed their boxes in our pantries.

Fake frooty artificial flavors can never match the oh-my-gosh life-changing-goodness of biting into a perfectly ripe melon or peach. No commercially-extruded "meat" burger or nugget will ever compare to the beauty of bison from my own ranch.

I may have left the family farm in Ohio years ago, but the farm has never left me. I still love to get my hands in the dirt and plant vegetables or fruit. I enjoy raising yaks, bison, camels for milk, quail for eggs, fruit trees, berries and muscadine grapes. Naturally, my wife, Suzie, and I love to see the delight on our children's faces when we serve them fresh kale, bison burgers, fruit smoothies or raspberry cobbler (which still isn't as good as my mom's).

TAKE BACK YOUR TASTE BUDS

Medical research not only shows how greasy, sweet, fast food destroys health; it is also extremely addictive. These foods "can hijack the brain in ways that resemble addictions to cocaine, nicotine and other drugs."[30] They program our brains to crave specific tastes and smells.

It's time we rediscover whole, natural and delicious foods. Everyone cannot revitalize the family farm like I did, but at least we can revolutionize our kitchens.

It's time we take back our taste buds. Since we were kids, our senses have been overwhelmed by great heaps of cheap, sweet, greasy, chemically-processed, flavor-enhanced, genetically-modified "food." Our foods are like a science project and we are the guinea pigs.

It is possible to break food addictions and retrain your senses. I know people who – at a more unhealthy time in their lives – couldn't stand the taste or feel of whole foods, or who hated pure, unadulterated water. These people retrained their taste buds by abstaining from the bad and eating the good. They used TIP (page 201) to reset their desires. Later when they tried the fake food again, they said, "Yuck! This stuff is gross!"

Give it a try. Try eating only the real deal for a month or two. You'll never go back, once your taste buds are reprogrammed to the awesomeness of

---

30   *Fatty Foods as Addictive as Cocaine*, www.bloomberg.com/news/2011-11-02/fatty-foods-addictive-as-cocaine-in-growing-body-of-science.html (January 2014).

real, whole foods as they were meant to be eaten. It's time you take back your taste buds!

OVERFED AND UNDERNOURISHED

Unlike impoverished nations and generations, we have plenty of food all year round. Still we are undernourished, lacking the life-giving essentials of real, whole foods, while killing ourselves with vast quantities of synthetic sweeteners, fats, additives, preservatives, genetically modified organisms, pesticides, herbicides, antibiotics and hormones.

> *Never eat more than you can lift.*
>
> — **Miss Piggy,**
> *The Muppet Show*

Overeating has contributed to an astronomical increase in obesity, diabetes, heart disease, stroke and cancer. "Two out of three adult Americans, and one out of three children between the ages of two and 19, are overweight or obese, according to the American Heart Association."[31] The Centers for Disease Control reports, "Childhood obesity has more than doubled in children and tripled in adolescents in the past 30 years."[32] About 600,000 Americans die of heart disease each year. "The number of people diagnosed with diabetes has risen from 1.5 million in 1958 to 18.8 million in 2010, an increase of epidemic proportions."[33] These numbers translate into more human sickness and personal suffering than any statistic can ever describe.

Western people are malnourished by high calorie, high chemical and low nutrient diets. Childhood obesity is perhaps the most tragic part of this epidemic. Researchers predict that children today can expect a shorter lifespan and poorer quality of life than their parents due to unhealthy choices.

Type 2 diabetes, once known as adult onset diabetes, is on the rise for people of all ages. According to the American Diabetes Association, "obesity is the hallmark of type 2 diabetes."[34] Its side effects include heart attack, stroke, blindness, amputation, kidney failure, nerve damage and liver disease. A 50-year-old person diagnosed with type 2 diabetes might

---

31   *Plant-Based Diet Extends Life Expectancy*, www.lamaruniversitypress.com/plant-based-diet-extends-life-expectancy-1.2975155#.UcnXbMqIWZE (January 2014).

32   *Childhood Obesity Facts*, www.cdc.gov/healthyyouth/obesity/facts.htm (January 2014).

33   *The Facts About Diabetes: A Leading Cause of Death in the U.S.*, http://ndep.nih.gov/diabetes-facts/ (January 2014).

34   *Type 2 Diabetes in Children*, www.childrenwithdiabetes.com/d_0n_d00.htm (January 2014).

have coronary bypass surgery at age 65, blindness at 75, and experience kidney failure and dialysis at 80.

Shockingly, obese children are now being diagnosed with type 2 diabetes. Imagine having type 2 diabetes at 15 and looking forward to – not a world of bright opportunities – but heart surgery, blindness, amputation, kidney failure and blood transfusions. Is this the death sentence we want for our children?

Break the trends by joining the Healing Revolution. Set yourself on the path to a long and fulfilling life by redefining and rediscovering amazing "real" food.

SUGAR, NOT FAT, MAKES YOU FAT

A common misconception is that eating fatty foods is the main cause of obesity. People often avoid fats while still consuming desserts, sweet drinks and diet drinks. Actually, sweeteners – both artificial and authentic – are the worst culprits when it comes to obesity.

While it is true that sugar has less calories per gram than fat, fats are more slowly assimilated into the body, causing a lingering feeling of being full. Sugar, on the other hand, is quickly turned to glucose, causing a sudden release of insulin to protect the body from sugar shock. This, in turn, makes you feel hungry again. It happens so quickly, in fact, that you may never feel as if your initial hunger has been satisfied.

So you eat more. In the end, people consistently eat higher quantities of sweets than fats to

The doctor of the future will give no medication, but will interest his patients in the care of the human frame, diet and in the cause and prevention of disease.

– Thomas Edison

satisfy hunger, which is why sugar makes you fat.[35] You are able to pack in much higher quantities of sweets than meats.

Surprisingly, artificial sweeteners are even worse, though they contain no calories. They trigger the pancreas to release insulin, which causes increased hunger, binge eating, obesity and the risk of diabetes. Research studies have linked these artificial sweeteners with greater weight gain, due to how the artificial sweeteners trick the body into storing every available calorie and increasing hunger.[36]

THE BEST AND WORST OF TIMES

Despite all the unhealthy aspects of food production today, there's also a bright side. New sustainable farming technologies are being used to improve the production of whole, healthy foods. Improved shipping technologies allow us to enjoy healthy fruits, vegetables, nuts, fish and meat from local and global markets in all seasons. Information on healthy food production and preservation is much more accessible to the average person, and the tools and materials are more easily obtained than in past decades.

Personally, I enjoy raising our own bison and putting up a little food from our garden and orchard at the end of the year. I love trading garden-fresh foods with our neighbors. Of course, food preservation at home is quite convenient thanks to the invention of the freezer and refrigerator. We also visit the farmer's markets whenever we can, to obtain locally grown, organic food. These markets may be the greatest, new-old healthy food idea we ever had.

The Healing Revolution is all about healthy choices. We possibly have more wholesome food choices today than at any time in history. But whether the good will outweigh the bad is a question that people must answer for themselves.

REFINERIES ARE FOR PETROLEUM, NOT FOOD

Some of the most destructive food production decisions in modern times have been made for cost and cosmetic reasons. People liked the color of white bread, so they bleached the flour. They liked the color of white sugar and white salt, so they super-refined them. They removed the bran

35   *Does sugar make you fat?*, www.obesity-info.com/2012/04/sugar-make-you-fat.html (January 2014).

36   *Saccharin and Aspartame, Compared with Sucrose, Induce Greater Weight Gain in Adult Wistar Rats*, www.sciencedirect.com/science/article/pii/S0195666312004138 (January 2014).

from rice and grains for a smoother texture. They created new kinds of fats and sugars in the laboratory, for reasons of taste, texture and profitability.

Natural, organically-grown, non-GMO (genetically modified organism), whole foods are much healthier than processed foods.[37] Unfortunately, plants and animals have been genetically modified to boost production and increase toleration to pesticides and herbicides that shouldn't be near our food in the first place! Worse yet, the pollen from genetically modified plants are contaminating natural crops, causing many farmers to wonder how they can possibly grow natural, unadulterated vegetables and grains in the coming years.

The sum effect of all these experiments upon humanity is lethal. It is shortening our lifespans. Our friends and neighbors are suffering and dying premature deaths because of these outrageous choices made to adulterate taste and increase financial gain. Refined foods provide empty calories that are void of what nature put in them. Empty calories leave us continually craving what we are missing, causing us to be overfed, undernourished and susceptible to disease.

Your body is genetically designed to live long and well on real, whole foods that are natural and unrefined. Eat whole grains. Avoid artificial sweeteners and processed foods. Eat honey and unrefined sweeteners. If it's white, don't bite!

TRY THIS!

MRT and TIP:
Healthy Desires
and Choices

(see Essential #8 for help using MRT and TIP)

- *Use Muscle Response Test (MRT) and Tap Into Potential (TIP) to strengthen healthy desires and choices.*
- *Use MRT to test statements like, "I <u>know</u> that is unhealthy. I <u>choose</u> instead. When I am tempted to make a bad choice, I will turn to a healthy choice. My desire <u>for</u> is increasing. I am excited about these new, healthy choices."*
- *Tap statements that are weak. Retest with MRT. Identify new statements that are most relevant to you.*
- *Repeat to strengthen healthy statements.*

---

37   *Research Sheds Light on Gluten Issues*, http://wholegrainscouncil.org/newsroom/blog/2012/01/research-sheds-light-on-gluten-issues (January 2014).

FEASTING, FASTING AND HUNGER

> *The more you eat, the less flavor; the less you eat, the more flavor.*
>
> *– Chinese Proverb*

The "Blue Zones" study that was mentioned earlier shows how the longest-living people on earth eat smaller portions of food than most Westerners. Western people like to eat, and food portion sizes are increasing all the time. People often graze all day like cows who have four stomachs, except that we only have one. As a consequence, our stomachs have become stretched and distended, which in turn leads to increased hunger and bigger food portions.

One problem is that many people confuse low blood sugar levels with hunger. The liver regulates sugar levels in the blood by storing up excess glucose after meals and by releasing it between meals. Too often people interrupt this natural process by feeding themselves at the slightest hint of a drop in blood sugar, which they mistakenly believe to be true hunger. So the liver, which was about to release stored glucose to keep the energy reserves flowing between meals, instead stores up more glucose. It's an unhealthy trap especially for people wanting to watch their weight.

I often advise people who think they might be hungry to drink water and get a short exercise burst, like a Two Minute Toning technique from the Fitness Chapter. That activates the liver to do its job of feeding the body, as it naturally should. I also recommend eating smaller meal portions: my personal preference is to have a protein shake in the morning and two light meals later in the day.

Fasting is another way to activate your body's natural metabolism, whether you skip one meal or a full day of meals. Giving your digestive system small breaks will make it stronger and keep you healthier. It is also a wonderful way for many of us who have never lacked food to learn that we are stronger than food and hunger, rather than giving food the power to run our lives. It brings a heightened sense of alertness and vitality. I encourage you to embrace hunger as a friend, not a foe.

BELLY FAT IS NOT JUST SKIN DEEP

Not all body fat is equal. "A big waistline puts you at increased risk for many health problems –– diabetes, heart disease, high blood pressure and stroke," according to Dr. Robert Eckel, president of the American Heart Association.[38] The National Institutes of Health states, "Excess fat in the stomach area is a greater risk factor for heart disease than excess fat in other parts of the body, such as on the hips."[39]

> *Leave your drugs in the chemist's pot if you can cure the patient with food.*
>
> *– Hippocrates*

The ugly truth about belly fat is that it is not just skin deep. Belly fat actually creeps deep inside the abdomen, coating the vital organs. It breaks down and finds its way into the blood stream and organs more easily than other fats, causing a chain reaction of problems such as increased bad cholesterol and triglycerides, high blood pressure, heart disease, high blood sugar and diabetes. One lethal effect of belly fat is metabolic syndrome, a high-risk combination of these conditions occurring concurrently. "Metabolic syndrome is becoming more common due to a rise in obesity rates among adults. In the future, metabolic syndrome may overtake smoking as the leading risk factor for heart disease."[40]

The following measurements indicate acceptable belly fat:

◆ *Waistline measurement divided by height should be less than .50. For example, a 5 foot 9 inch (69 inch) person with a 36 inch waist has too much belly fat. (36 ÷ 69 = .52)*
◆ *Waistline measurement divided by hip measurement should be less than .85 (women) or .90 (men). For example, a 30 inch waist and a 36 inch hip is acceptable. (30 ÷ 36 = .83)*
◆ *In general, waistline measurement should be less than 35 inches (women) or 40 inches (men). This is not as accurate as the other measurements, since it does not take body size into account.*

---

38   *The Risks of Belly Fat*, www.webmd.com/diet/features/the-risks-of-belly-fat (January 2014).
39   *What is Metabolic Syndrome?* www.nhlbi.nih.gov/health/health-topics/topics/ms/ (January 2014).
40   Ibid.

One natural way to control belly fat is to eat a healthy diet of whole foods. Moreover, stress is directly linked to belly fat. For some wonderful suggestions about reducing stress, see the chapters about the Human Spirit, Fitness, Sleep, Nature and Hands On Techniques. Belly fat is also a common sign of adrenal problems; 80 to 90 percent of my patients with excessive belly fat had adrenal fatigue or dysfunction. See Essential #8, Hands On Techniques, for the Ragland's Test that is a sure indicator of adrenal issues.

See www.DrFrankKing.com for a free Whole Health Appraisal that can help you identify potential causes of belly fat. Additionally, to shrink your stomach size and help control your appetite, see the HOT Essential Chapter for a unique tool I developed for my patients.

SOME HEALTHY RECOMMENDATIONS

If you'd like to make some healthy nutritional changes but you're not sure where to start, here are a few recommendations:

> *Let food be your medicine and medicine be your food.*
>
> *—Hippocrates*

- ◆ *Eat plenty of natural plants and animals: uncanned, unprocessed and organic if possible.*
- ◆ *Go wild! Wild-based plants and animals have healing qualities that connect us with our root genetics, restoring inner health. That's why I like eating wild foods like bison, yak, camel's milk, herbs, muscadine grapes and other wild foods.*
- ◆ *Eat real, whole foods. You will avoid many common illnesses by simply eating natural, whole foods. The closer it is to the earth or sea from which it came, the more whole it is.*
- ◆ *Before you consume a questionable food or beverage, stop and ask yourself, "Is this really good for me?" Your healthy instinct might add years to your life (and life to your years) by exposing bad choices.*
- ◆ *Eat whole, unrefined sea salt. It is a powerhouse of about 80 minerals that are not found in refined salt. These minerals are good for your whole body, including your cardiovascular system.*
- ◆ *Read ingredient labels. Do not eat food products unless all of the ingredients are great for your health.*
- ◆ *Chew more. Studies show that people who chew their food up to 40 times per bite eat smaller portions than those who chew 15 times. Obese*

*people chew less, eat faster and eat more.[41] Better chewing liquefies
the food with digestive factors in your saliva, improving digestion. It
also slows the meal down, giving the brain more time to learn that your
stomach is full.*

◆ *Eat the rainbow. The Standard American Diet (SAD) of meat, potatoes
and baked goods is bland and colorless. The refining process removes
color, vitamins and more. Nature packs intense nutrition in super-colored
foods like red peppers, yellow squash, orange citrus, leafy greens,
blueberries, grapes, eggplants and rainbow-colored tomatoes or carrots.
Colorful foods have more essential vitamins, enzymes, anti-oxidants and
a power-packed array of phytonutrients. For example, red, yellow and
orange carotenoids help fight disease because of their strong anti-oxidant
characteristics.*

◆ *Think of food as medicine. The rainbow foods, for example, are high
in essential nutrients like carotenoids, flavonoids, potassium, fiber,
vitamins A, B, C and E. They super-charge your body with the potential to
overcome the worst diseases that cripple men, women and children who
are on the SAD diet. Real food gives you more energy, helps you think
clearer and keeps you disease-free.*

◆ *Retrain your tastes. You just might develop a passion for the healthy foods
you despised as a child. Epigenetics proves that you can reshape your genetic
expression, and as you do, you can also change your taste preferences.*

◆ *Rethink your priorities. A shopping bag full of healthy food may cost you a
few bucks more. But if you had a serious illness, you'd pay any price to be
healed. You will pay a big price for eating the empty calories of junk food.
Think of the extra cost now as an investment in fabulous health. In the
end, healthy choices will be cheaper and a lot less painful.*

◆ *Start simply. If your budget does not allow you to make big changes yet,
buy cheaper whole foods like legumes and whole grains (for example,
brown rice, beans, quinoa and lentils). Watch for sale prices on organic,
whole, healthy foods. Locate some nearby discount health food stores.*

◆ *Eat foods that are in season where you live. Local foods are healthier and
more affordable when in season.*

◆ *Freeze, bottle or can. Some of the tastiest, healthiest food is dirt cheap
when in season. Put some away, however you can, for later in the year.*

---

41   Jie Li et al., " Improvement in chewing activity reduces energy intake," *The American Journal of Clinical Nutrition*, September
2011, vol. 94, no. 3, 709-716.

- Enjoy fermented foods. Fermentation is the most ancient and natural way to preserve foods. It also makes foods more digestible by breaking down cellulose that the human body can't normally digest. Fermented foods are a regular part of the Blue Zones diet, where people live longest.
- Fermented foods include sauerkraut, kimchee, yogurt, kefir, certain cheeses, apple cider vinegar, balsamic vinegar, wine, sourdough bread, fermented pickles, kombucha, tempeh, miso and naturally fermented soy sauce.
- Buy organic fruits and vegetables. See the "Dirty Dozen" list that follows this section. Here is a simple rule of thumb: It is especially important to buy organic if you're going to eat the skin of the fruit or vegetable.
- Buy organic and grass-fed meats when you can. Look for wild-caught fish, not farm fish. Choose organic, free-range, hormone- and antibiotic-free meat and poultry and eggs.
- Buy organic dairy products. Whey is one of my favorite forms of protein and it can be added to soups and smoothies.
- Here's an interesting generalization about grocery stores: Most of the unhealthy, processed food is in the inner isles. Shop the perimeter of the store for whole foods like produce, meats and dairy. Dive into the inner isles for grains, legumes, oils, nuts and a few other real foods.
- Vary your diet. Most people eat the same 20 foods over and over again. This can trigger food allergies or sensitivities. Avoid these problems by rotating foods and giving the most common ones a rest. Dinnertime can be an adventure when you put a few new grains, legumes and vegetables on the table.
- Plant a garden. Start small and expand it a little each year as you learn what plants grow best in your soil. Plant fruit trees and berry vines. You will taste the amazing difference in freshly-picked produce.
- Raise chickens for eggs. Poultry is well-adapted to life in all climates, in the city (where allowed) or in the country. They are surprisingly easy to maintain. Fresh eggs are a delightful addition to a healthy diet. Personally, I'd rather awaken to a rooster's crow than an alarm clock.[42]
- If you are new to nutrition, Harvard Medical School's Healthy Eating Plate will give you a good, general picture of a balanced diet, which should include fresh vegetables and fruits complimented with whole grains and healthy protein.[43]

---

[42] For practical help gardening, raising animals or more, see Carla Emery, *The Encyclopedia of Country Living* (Seattle: Sasquatch Books) or the *Whole Earth Catalog* and family of publications (www.wholeearth.com/index.php) (January 2014).

[43] *Healthy Eating Plate vs. USDA's MyPlate*, www.hsph.harvard.edu/nutritionsource/healthy-eating-plate-vs-usda-myplate/ (January 2014).

- Fast from all foods or simply eliminate one type of food for short periods of time. Skip just one meal, if that's all you want to do. The amazing benefits of fasting include cleansing, detoxification, rest for the digestive system, enhanced ability to fight disease, increased mental clarity, increased energy and inner stillness. Hunger is too powerful of a force in our lives. We become slaves to food. Put hunger in its place by saying, "You can wait. My life, health and happiness are more important than food." This brings an incredible sense of freedom.[44]

- Involve the whole family. Make healthy choices for your kids. Put them in charge of shopping for one food group in the supermarket. Get them excited about healthy cooking, gardening, farmer's markets, or picking fruits or berries from orchards. Find an organic farm or dairy that gives tours. Too many kids don't have a clue where their food comes from.[45]

- The average child sees about 10,000 junk food advertisements per year, which is probably more than they hear from you about healthy choices. Share this book with your family. Help them to get excited about healthy living, but avoid preaching.

- Never nag or condemn your friends, co-workers or extended family for their choices. If you disagree, do what you know is right for yourself and keep the focus on yourself. Keep a positive attitude and show (more than tell) others how healthy living can make life better.

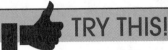

TRY THIS!

MRT: Foods and Supplements

MRT is explained on page 197.

- Diversity applies to digestion as much as to any other human quality. Use Muscle Response Test (MRT) to determine which foods, supplements, vitamins, minerals and herbs are good for you.

- Look at ingredients lists. Run more tests and compare notes to determine which item(s) you are intolerant of in a complex list of ingredient.

---

44   The Benefits of Fasting, www.allaboutfasting.com/benefits-of-fasting.html (January 2014).

45   I was shocked to watch "Jamie Oliver's Food Revolution" where first graders were unable to identify common vegetables like tomato, potato, cauliflower and eggplant. See: www.youtube.com/watch?v=bGYs4KS_djg (January 2014).

WHERE THE WILD THINGS ARE

Wild plants are among the most nutrient-rich foods on the planet. Moreover, you don't have to travel far to find them. They are likely growing in your yard. Search online for photos and descriptions of local edible plants such as lamb's quarter, milk thistle, plantain, salad burnet, dandelion leaves, violet flowers, nasturtiums, grape leaves and chicory. Pick these, wash them and nibble on them. Make a tossed salad and flavor it with healthy salad dressing. Ask the locals where to find wild blackberries, raspberries, blueberries, elderberries and mulberries. Don't eat anything that grows beside highways, power plants, factories, refineries or high traffic areas where pollutants contaminate the plants. Harvest watercress from clear, running streams.

The Environmental Working Group's
DIRTY DOZEN List of Fruits and Vegetables

The Environmental Working Group, Executive Summary, www.ewg.org/foodnews/summary.php (January 2014). This list is constantly updated, so check the website for the latest version.

DIRTY DOZEN (most important to buy organic)	CLEAN FIFTEEN (least important to buy organic)
Apple	Asparagus
Celery	Avocado
Cherry tomatoes	Cabbage
Cucumber	Cantaloupe
Grapes	Sweet corn
Hot peppers	Eggplant
Nectarines (imported)	Grapefruit
Peaches	Kiwi
Potatoes	Mangos
Spinach	Mushrooms
Strawberries	Onions
Sweet Bell Peppers	Papayas
Kale/Collard Green	Pineapples
Summer Squash	Sweet peas (frozen)
	Sweet Potatoes

VITAMINS AND SUPPLEMENTS

I am a big advocate of vitamins, herbs and supplements, having used them personally and with my patients for many years. But not everything labeled "vitamin" is beneficial to your body.

For example, most vitamin C tablets do not contain what your body really needs. Many years ago, researchers looked for the reasons why citrus fruit cured scurvy in sailors. They isolated ascorbic acid, which many people consider to be synonymous with vitamin C. In reality, ascorbic acid is merely one component of the vitamin C complex, which also contains rutin, bioflavonoids, factor K, factor J, factor P, tyrosinase and ascorbinogen. It is interesting to note that researchers found that potatoes, which include a very small amount of complex vitamin C with all components included, are more effective in curing scurvy than large dosages of pure ascorbic acid.

The same is true with all vitamins. Most substances that are sold as vitamins are in fact isolates (isolated from the complete, complex vitamin components). Most people buy these vitamin isolates because they are cheap and easy to obtain. These chemically-synthesized isolates are not nearly as effective as the natural, complex vitamins.

Your best solution is to obtain nutritional supplements from organic, whole food sources. Use the MRT to determine what nutritional supplements will be best for your unique health needs. Re-test regularly since your body's needs change.

General Vitamin Recommendations

▷ **Multi-Vitamin:** *Most people can benefit from a complex, whole-food based multi-vitamin.*

▷ **Vitamin D3:** *Especially important in winter and times of low sun exposure.*

▷ **Fish and plant oils:** *The Omega-3s in fish and plant oils and certain wild foods reduces inflammation that leads to chronic conditions like cancer, asthma, cardiovascular disease and rheumatoid arthritis. To avoid consuming heavy metals like mercury, avoid fish oil from carnivorous fish higher in the food chain.*

HERBS AND SUPERFOODS

Many herbs taste good when eaten alone. Others are delicious sprinkled on salads or dishes. It's a matter of taste, so do some research and use MRT to discover which herbs are most beneficial for your health. A few of the many natural herbs and superfoods that can enhance your health include:

- **Jujube date.** *Eliminates excess mucous, strengthens digestion and circulation, and relieves stress.*
- **Licorice.** *Coats the stomach lining and calms indigestion and heartburn.*
- **Foti root.** *Helps detoxify the body and rejuvenate nerves, brain cells and endocrine glands.*
- **Goji berries.** *Traditionally used for anti-aging purposes; helps to avoid diabetes, high blood pressure and fever.*
- Cordyceps and reishi mushrooms. *Boosts immune system; helps avoid cancers.*
- **Aloe vera.** *Soothes skin irritations, burns and sunburn; taken orally for arthritis pain and irritable bowels.*
- **Curcumin.** *Helps relieve minor pain symptoms; is a natural anti-inflammatory.*
- **Maca root.** *Normalizes hormonal imbalance and increases sex drive.*
- **Kelp, spirulina, blue green algae, micro algae, chlorella and other seaweeds.** *Great detoxifiers and sources of minerals including iodine. Kelp is a good source of vitamin B12.*
- **Hemp seeds.** *Contains all 20 amino acids; high in Omega-3 fatty acids; promotes healthy muscles.*
- **Bee pollen.** *One of nature's most nourishing superfoods; used for anti-aging and to promote healing.*
- **Camu-camu berry.** *Contains concentrated natural vitamin C for mental clarity, immune system strengthening and collagen production for healthy joints and skin.*
- **Elderberry.** *Helps fight fungal, bacterial and viral infections; strengthens the immune system.*
- **Muscadine grapes.** *Contains 40 times more phytonutrients than traditional grapes; contains antioxidants.*
- **Schizandra berries.** *Rejuvenates kidneys and sex glands; helps relieve stress and fatigue.*
- **Camel's milk.** *Studies have shown it to be helpful for autism, hepatitis, some cancers and anti-aging.*

VEGETARIANS, VEGANS, PESCATARIANS, CARNIVORES, OMNIVORES AND MORE

People are so incredibly diverse in their dietary needs. Nobody can claim that one diet such as vegetarian, vegan, pescatarian or carnivore is "best" for everybody. You can, however, determine what is best for you, for this particular time of life.

For example, I was a vegetarian for most of my 20s – quite a feat, considering that I was raised on a beef farm. My diet suited me well for a while, but gradually my body and mind began to weaken. I had low blood pressure, fatigue and poor concentration. My cholesterol and triglycerides tested too low. My saliva was too alkaline. Simply put, I felt terrible.

Then I had a vision of a Great Horned Buffalo riding across the prairie to rescue me from starvation. Just kidding. Still, it was a bison that "saved" me. I had opposed red meat primarily because of the unhealthy nature of most conventional beef and pork, and because of the inhumane practices used in the meat industry. Then I learned about the health benefits of game meats and naturally-raised bison. I discovered that research highlighting the negative aspects of red meat pointed to unhealthy *beef* production, not to game meat or the leaner, naturally-raised bison. So I added bison to my diet. Within a few days my physical and mental capacities returned in full. I've been loving healthy, wild, red meat ever since that day.

Every person's needs are different, but I have known many patients who are like me when I was a vegetarian, who perhaps ate some fish or poultry. They reacted negatively to red meat, until they tried eating natural bison or other wild meats. Many of them found that adding healthy red meat to their diet made them feel better and increased their functionality, which only strengthens my opposition to unhealthy meats.

Your nutritional needs may change in time. You may want to try going meat-free for a period of time, as I did. A vegetarian diet was appropriate for me for a while and perhaps it helped detoxify my body. But after several years, my body began to cry out for meat. Similarly, your needs may change in time.

Mainly, no one diet applies to everybody. We are diverse human beings and biological individuality is as unique as our fingerprints. One person's best meal could be another person's worst.

DIET VS. LIVE-IT

I am opposed to diets that consist of giving up unhealthy foods for a period of time in order to lose weight, after which the unhealthy foods are once more consumed. It is better to improve your lifetime habits. Why diet when you can live-it? Healthy nutrition is an ongoing lifestyle. Change your habits and your preferences for life.

See my website, www. DrFrankKing.com, for helpful articles and videos about healthy nutrition. Additionally, I have included some tools for improving your health in Essential #8: Hands On Techniques, including an amazing technique for manually shrinking the size of your stomach and thereby returning your food volume and caloric intake to a more natural level. This unique technique could change your life.

You may be able to determine what diet is best for you as I did years ago, by observing how your body responds to different food types. The Hands On Techniques chapter explains how to monitor your ileocecal valve for food toxicities, sensitivities or intolerances. You can take a doctor-administered food allergy blood test, or even better, try the Muscle Response Test (MRT).

Glycemic Index

The glycemic index (GI) is a scale of 0 to 100 describing the rise in blood sugar after eating a standard portion of carbohydrates. Foods with a high GI (e.g., white sugar (65) or white bread (89)) are quickly digested, causing a swift rise in blood sugar and insulin. Foods with a low GI (e.g., peanuts (13) or carrots (16)) are slowly digested, causing a gradual rise in blood sugar and a delay in hunger. Whole foods have a lower GI. Foods with higher GI cause fast digestion, increased hunger and greater weight gain.

A helpful glycemic index search tool is provided by the University of Sydney's GI Group: **www.glycemicindex.com/.**

TAKE BACK YOUR KITCHEN

Once upon a time, modern people trusted the experts to tell them what was good and healthy to eat. They trusted somebody else to watch over their diet, their kitchens, their nutritional health and the nutritional health of their children.

Today the question is, who can you trust to make your nutritional health decision?

Can you trust advertisers, marketers, agri-executives, food researchers, or genetic engineers? Can you trust governmental agencies? The United States Department of Agriculture (USDA) is both in charge of promoting agriculture as well as monitoring food safety and warning consumers of potential dangers. Do you see a conflict of interest there?

Who can you trust? The so-called "experts," or your own instincts, your best judgment and what you have learned to be true for you?

I think you know who you can trust.

Let us stand shoulder to shoulder. Let us rise up and take back our kitchens.

Let us live long and prosper by joining the Healing Revolution.

SELF-EVALUATION
NUTRITION

My Life-Destroying Choices *(e.g.: too much sugar and white flour, lack of protein and minerals, too many processed foods)*	**My Life-Affirming Choices** *(e.g.: desire healthy, whole, natural foods, try new foods and stop eating bad foods)*
1	1
2	2
3	3
4	4
5	5
6	6
7	7

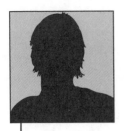

My Story:
Dr. Wicked Hand

I had some serious problems when I was five years old. In fact, I was so weak and frail that my parents were worried that I might not survive. They took me to several doctors and the best they could guess was that I might have leukemia. I was tired and lethargic all the time. I couldn't put any meat on my skinny bones.

Out of desperation, Mom and Dad took me to a foreign doctor who, I'm told, had a sketchy reputation. Nevertheless, he was known to be successful with some of the more unusual cases. He practiced medicine out of a single-wide home in a trailer park near our farm. His name was Dr. Wickenham, but all the kids just called him Dr. Wicked Hand.

This unconventional doctor quickly determined that I had food allergies. I remember that one of the items he told me to stop eating was ketchup, which didn't make me happy since that happened to be my favorite "vegetable."

My parents changed my diet and I began to experience results. My energy returned and I was able, for the first time, to run and play and keep up with the other kids. I gained confidence and became more competitive.

I remember playing football and receiving a kick-off. I charged into a dozen kids like a mad rhino, breaking through the pack with speed I'd never experienced before, making a glorious touchdown.

I'm as good as they are, I thought. *Maybe even better.*

Soon I was baling hay and picking rocks out of the fields with my brothers and my dad. I felt like a new person. I'm glad my parents stepped outside of mainstream medicine to find the remedy I needed. I'm also grateful for Dr. Wicked Hand who did for me what no other doctor could.

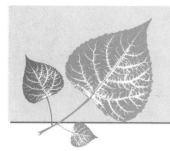

ESSENTIAL #3:
WATER

A merchant sold pills that had been invented to quench thirst. You need only swallow one pill a week, and you would feel no need of anything to drink.

"Why are you selling those?" asked the little prince.

"Because they save a tremendous amount of time," said the merchant. "Computations have been made by experts. With these pills, you save fifty-three minutes in every week."

"And what do I do with those fifty-three minutes?"

"Anything you like ..."

"As for me," said the little prince to himself, "if I had fifty-three minutes to spend as I liked, I should walk at my leisure toward a spring of fresh water."

– Antoine de Saint-Exupéry,
The Little Prince

After hiking ten hours in 100-degree heat without drinking any water, Dave Buschow fell face-down in the Utah desert. He died of dehydration less than 100 yards from his destination: a cave with a pool of water.

Dave Buschow's 11 hiking companions told reporters that he was experiencing cramps, his speech was slurred and he was hallucinating so badly that he mistook a tree for a person. Nevertheless, the leaders of the wilderness-survival expedition who accompanied Dave didn't offer any of the emergency water that they carried. This survival program encouraged participants to push themselves to their limits and beyond.

Apparently Dave Buschow, who died July 17, 2006, at the age of 29, discovered his limits.[46]

---

46   *Hiker Dies Of Thirst With Water All Around*, www.cbsnews.com/2100-501843_162-2757021.html (January 2014).

DEHYDRATION

Next to oxygen, water is the most vital substance for survival on earth. The healthy human body is about 70 percent water – similar to the percentage of water on the earth's surface. Water is not only good for life; it is essential for survival.

> *Thousands have lived without love, not one without water.*
>
> *– 20th century Anglo-American Poet W.H. Auden*

Many people are dehydrated and they don't know it, having scaly skin, dry nose and dry mouth. People who do not respond to the little voice inside that cries "I'm thirsty" eventually shrivel and shrink. In the extreme, their flesh and organs turn to jerky. Dehydration leads to premature aging. I have seen chronically dehydrated people whose skin looked much older than it should. But I have also seen well-hydrated seniors with youthful skin.

Bodily fluids need constant flow and motion to remain healthy and pure. Dehydration leads to stagnation and water retention, as the body fights to hold onto its fluids at all costs. The toxins that are normally flushed downstream are trapped when the body becomes dehydrated, causing a dangerous increase in toxicity. A dehydrated body is like a stagnant pond with leaches, slimy scum and the smell of death. A hydrated person, on the other hand, is like a beautiful mountain meadow flowing with fresh, crystal streams.

Your body's "thirst indicator" is designed to warn you that the pure streams are getting polluted. It's similar to the gas gauge on your car, although for many people thirst is not so much like the needle that indicates how full the tank is. For them, thirst is more like the red warning light that comes on just before running out of gas. That sensation of thirst is a sign of dehydration.

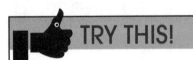

TRY THIS!

MRT: Test for Dehydration

MRT is explained on page 197.

- *While your healing buddy tests your strong muscle, pull a tuft of hair on your head, not quite to the point of pain.*
- *If you are dehydrated, your muscle will go weak.*
- *Drink pure spring or well water and repeat the test. Your muscle will likely remain strong.*

"By the time you get thirsty, you will have lost energy from the water that you should have drunk ... before you get thirsty," says Dr. Fereydoon Batmanghelidj, author of *Water for Health, for Healing, for Life*. "If you don't allow the gas tank of your car to [run out] before you stop and get some gas, then why should you let your body become thirsty so that it stalls on the roadside before you drink water?"[47]

Your body needs water all day long ... *before* the red light starts to show.

THREE SIMPLE AT-HOME TESTS FOR DEHYDRATION

♦ *Urine color:* Urine may be deep yellow when you awake in the morning. Otherwise it should be clear to pale yellow. Darker urine is a sign of dehydration. (Unless you are taking "B" complex vitamins; then your urine will be more yellow.)

♦ *Skin pinch test:* Pinch the skin on the back of your hand and hold for three seconds. Release. The ridge from the pinch should be gone in less than a second; otherwise you are likely dehydrated.

♦ *Tongue test:* Take your index finger and rub the center of your tongue. It should feel smooth, like wet wax paper. If it feels rough, you are dehydrated.

YOU ARE THIRSTY, NOT HUNGRY

People often confuse hunger with thirst. From childhood they are taught to fill their mouths with milk, sweets, snacks or anything but water when the feeling of need hits the stomach. Many times when that feeling comes, the body is simply saying, "I'm thirsty."

Nutritionist Dr. Gabriel Cousens says, "When you start to hydrate by drinking enough water, then your appetite goes down because you're actually fulfilling your body's needs – which is water. And that's also a very powerful way to lose weight, but also, in a sense, the hydration makes everything – including your brain – work a lot better."[48]

Too many people have lost the taste for water so they reach for a sweet drink, a candy bar or a fried comfort food. The result is that we have become a generation of dehydrated heavyweights. We are now empowered to take back our water.

47   *Water Cure: An Interview with Dr. Batmanghelidj*, www.naturalnews.com/Report_water_cure_7.html (January 2014).

48   *Gabriel Cousens In-Depth Interview: Eating Live, Raw Food*, http://fashiontribes.typepad.com/main/2005/06/untitled_podcas_5.html (January 2014).

DRINK, DRINK, DRINK

Every cell in your body is like that guy in the desert, dying for a drink. A good rule of thumb is to drink at least half your body weight in ounces of water each day. For example, if you weigh 160 pounds, drink 80 ounces of water per day. That's 10 one-cup glasses.

If you don't care for the taste of pure, spring or well water, try mixing a teaspoon of sea salt into a quart or liter of water. Experiment with different concentrations according to your taste preferences.

If you have been consistently under-hydrated, you may complain about having to urinate frequently after raising your water consumption. This reaction is temporary and natural. Your body has been retaining water to keep cells from dying, even though the water was polluted. Drink smaller quantities of water more often – perhaps four ounces every thirty minutes or so – rather than guzzling huge quantities at one time. This will retrain your body to keep its fluid levels healthy and happy. When you get together with your healing buddies, ask each other how you've been doing with your water consumption.

I, too, have struggled to stay hydrated. I have posted "DRINK!" signs around the home and office, just to keep me on track. I leave water bottles in many different places so it's never inconvenient for me to drink.

Sweating is a wonderful, natural detoxification process that improves physiological functions and beautifies the skin and organs. It provides one more escape for the sludge in your body. I strongly recommend working out hard enough to break into sweat, several times a week. Naturally, drink more water than usual when you sweat.

THE REAL THING?

I once had a patient named Barb who liked to drink diet cola – up to eight cans a day.

That's a lot of aspartame, phosphoric acid and phenylalanine to pump into your body, I thought.

"Why do you drink so much diet cola?" I asked Barb.

"It tastes good," she said, "and it has zero calories."

I tried to explain to her the harmful risks associated with diet soft drinks, such as kidney failure, metabolic syndrome, diabetes, reproductive system damage and bone loss. I told her about how artificial sweeteners like saccharin and aspartame actually cause higher weight gain than sugar because of how the body stores fat after being "tricked" by artificial sweeteners. (See the Nutrition Essential chapter for more information about that issue.)

After our discussion, Barb quit drinking diet cola. Within a few weeks she lost five stubborn pounds ... just by kicking the can! After a month I saw Barb in my office again.

"Are you still abstaining from diet cola?" I asked.

"To tell you the truth, Dr. King, I nearly fell off the bandwagon. I'd been thinking a lot about how I just wanted one more taste of diet cola. Then when I had the opportunity to pop the top, I did it."

"So ... what happened?" I asked.

"I took one sip and then I spit it right out. I couldn't believe how terrible it tasted! All I could taste were those yucky chemicals in my mouth. It was awful!"

"That's amazing, Barb. And this is the same cola you had been drinking all the time?"

She nodded. "It's the same old cola, so I guess I'm the one that's changed. Maybe I liked it then because my taste buds were numbed by drinking it all the time. But not anymore. Not after a month of doing without. One thing I know for sure, Dr. King, is that I'll never drink diet cola again."

> *The mystery of language was revealed to me. I knew then that 'W-A-T-E-R' meant the wonderful cool something that was flowing over my hand. That living word awakened my soul, gave it light, joy, set it free.*
>
> *– Helen Keller,*
> *The Story of*
> *My Life*

People who drink just one serving of soda a day increase their risk of diabetes by 22 percent.[49] But the health risks of all the unnatural chemicals in diet sodas may even be more serious than the sweeteners in other drinks.

Pure, natural water is the real thing.

---

49   *Just One Soda Increases Your Risk of Diabetes by 22 Percent*, www.foxnews.com/health/2013/04/25/just-one-soda-increases-your-risk-diabetes-by-22-percent/ (January 2014).

TECHNOLOGICAL ADVANCES
IN BEVERAGE ENGINEERING

> *Our bodies are*
> *molded rivers.*
>
> *— 18th century*
> *German*
> *Philosopher*
> *Novalis*

Technological advances in beverage engineering have made it possible for people to go from cradle to grave without taking one sip of life-giving water, if they so choose. Literally. Diapered consumers start with infant formula, which is soon replaced by pasteurized milk. After that, the cocktail selection multiplies rapidly with the addition of chocolate milk, strawberry milk, juice boxes, soft drinks, sports drinks, electrolyte-replacement drinks, coffee, tea, beer, wine, alcohol coolers and many more options. Seniors are even given nutritional beverages, something of which their great-grandparents ¬— who lived more healthy lives — never dreamed.

One of the most common ingredients in drinks these days is high fructose corn syrup (HFCS). HFCS is manufactured by using enzymes to convert much of the glucose in corn syrup to fructose, which tastes sweeter than plain sugar. HFCS is very quickly digested and turned into fat, making it a primary cause of obesity.

"HFCS also increases uric acid levels, further increasing the risk of diabetes, high blood pressure, kidney disease and obesity," says Dr. Richard Johnson, author of *The Sugar Fix: The High Fructose Fallout That Is Making You Fat and Sick*.[50]

It's difficult to determine what is worse for you: sugar, high fructose corn syrup, artificial sweeteners, artificial colorants, artificial flavors, phosphorous additives in soft drinks, or any of the other harmful chemicals in the wide assortments of water substitutes that fill our cups, bottles and mouths today.

Read the ingredients on everything that goes in your mouth. Many so-called health drinks or juice drinks contain HFCS. Even if a drink is pure juice, it contains a large quantity of fructose. Compare grams of sugar per serving, and you will find that some juices have more sugar than soft drinks. It takes several pieces of fruit to make one glass of juice. I doubt if you would typically eat that much fruit in one sitting. Consider grabbing a glass of water

---

50   Richard Johnson, *The Sugar Fix: The High Fructose Fallout That Is Making You Fat and Sick* (New York: Pocket Books, 2008).

Everywhere water is a thing of beauty, gleaming in the dewdrops; singing in the summer rain; shining in the ice-gems till the leaves all seem to turn to living jewels; spreading a golden veil over the setting sun; or a white gauze around the midnight moon.

**– John Ballantine Gough,
A Glass of Water**

and a piece of fruit instead, to lower your sugar intake and increase the natural fiber, which is great for your gut.

As explained earlier in the Nutrition Chapter, sugar, more than fat, makes you fat. It's not easy to break an addiction to sugar, HFCS or artificial sweeteners. It may mean retraining your senses to the refreshing taste of delicious water with the help of TIP (see the chapter on Hands On Techniques), but once you break the bad habit, your body will repay you with health benefits that no beverage company on earth could ever manufacture.

DIURETICS

Contrary to reason, many drinks actually dry you up because they contain diuretics. Diuretics inhibit the kidney's role in reabsorbing water and salt, causing excessive urination.

Caffeine and alcohol are the most common diuretics. Studies show that the more alcohol you drink, the more difficult it becomes to retain water. Alcohol-induced dehydration also causes a deficiency of nutrients and minerals such as magnesium, potassium, calcium and zinc.

Excessive alcohol consumption is never healthy, but a glass of wine a day may actually be good for you. Many of the longest-living people on earth drink a little wine each day, and nearly all of them drink life-giving spring water. If you drink coffee or tea, buy only organic products to avoid the toxic chemicals used in non-organic food production. Additionally, drink plenty of pure water to counteract the diuretic effects of caffeinated tea or coffee.

Caffeinated soft drinks, energy drinks and specialty drinks with names like caramel-mocha-latte-espresso-supreme have off-the-chart quantities of sugar or HFCS. Add whipped cream and you're getting around 500 calories – enough for a whole meal, although these calories have almost no nutritional value. They are the kind of calories that build flabby bodies. That sweet drink will give you a quick buzz and soon lead you back for more when the fatigue of a low blood sugar crash returns.

SLOW DEATH BY DEHYDRATION

Dr. Fereydoon Batmanghelidj was a political prisoner in Iran's infamous Evin Prison during the Iranian Revolution from 1979 to 1983. When asked to help a fellow prisoner who was suffering with peptic ulcer pain, the only remedy Dr. Batmanghelidj could obtain was water. Dr. Batmanghelidj gave the man two glasses of water and within eight minutes his pain disappeared. The patient remained pain-free for the rest of his imprisonment by drinking two glasses of water every three hours. Dr. Batmanghelidj successfully treated 3,000 suffering prisoners using water alone. He conducted additional research into water's effectiveness in treating and preventing degenerative diseases. When offered an early release, Dr. Batmanghelidj decided to stay an extra four months to complete his research.

Astronauts living on the International Space Station will get their drinking water from a new system that recycles their urine into drinkable water. Said one space station astronaut, "It would have been nice to get a heads-up on that before we got here."

— actor and author Seth Meyers

It's a good thing he stayed, because his findings revealed that the remarkable glass of water that you hold in your hands has more power to determine your fate – for good or for bad – than you might imagine. According to Dr. Batmanghelidj, dehydration is a major contributing factor to chronic diseases such as:[51]

▶ **Asthma and allergies.** Research suggest that drinking more water minimizes asthma and allergy symptoms. Water is lost through the process of breathing. The body conserves water by releasing histamine into the air passages, which constricts air and helps retain water. Histamine production decreases when water intake is increased.

---

51   Fereydoon Batmanghelidj, *Your Body's Many Cries for Water* (Falls Church, VA: Global Health Solutions, Inc., 1998).

▶ **Obesity**. As mentioned earlier, people often confuse hunger and thirst. A well-hydrated belly is more satisfied, not always shouting for food. Ample water is also needed for the liver to cleanse the body. Dehydrated livers lead to higher levels of fat storage.

▶ **Diabetes.** Type 2 diabetes, the kind that once only hit older people, is now common among obese teenagers. The rise in diabetes is directly related to increased obesity, which in turn may be linked to not drinking enough water.

▶ **Heart disease**. When the body senses that too much liquid is being removed from the cells, it produces more cholesterol to "plug the gaps" in the cell wall. This has the negative consequence of clogging the arteries with cholesterol, constricting the blood flow and heightening the risk of heart attack.

▶ **High blood pressure and stroke**. Dehydration causes constriction of the capillaries to compensate for the lower liquid volume. This in turn increases arterial pressure, which can cause strokes. Moreover, dehydration can also lead to dangerously low blood pressure.

▶ **Stress and depression.** Brain signals in a dehydrated brain are inhibited. This imbalance of neurotransmitters in the brain can lead to stress and depression.

▶ **Digestive disorders.** Belly pain is a common thirst reaction. Dehydration contributes to heartburn, indigestion, acid reflux, colitis, hiatal hernia and ulcers. Adequate water is necessary for the mucous membranes to create a natural barrier against stomach acid.

▶ **Musculoskeletal pain.** Dehydration causes pain by shrinking the cushioning cartilage and discs between joints and vertebrae. These healthy "pillows" shrink with age. Proper hydration can help maintain their youthful form and function.

▶ **Headaches.** Headaches are one of the common symptoms of dehydration. Proactively drink four ounces of water every 30 minutes to head off headaches.

THE BEST WATER

No water is as good for you as fresh, clean, spring water. The earth receives the rain and filters it, then it mineralizes and revitalizes it. Living water ripens in the earth's womb and is finally birthed to the surface as mature, spring water. It is living, flowing and naturally charged with the minerals you need.

If possible, locate a pure spring and fill up your own glass bottles. Second to that, consider buying bottled spring water. Well water may be healthy, although it is not "mature," not having experienced the full mineralization and purification processes of rising naturally to the surface. It also may be contaminated by local mining, farming or manufacturing activity, so have your well water thoroughly tested.

Read the label carefully on any water you buy. Bottled spring water is best. Both distilled water and reverse osmosis (RO) water have been stripped of their essential minerals. Water that says "filtered" is often reverse osmosis water. Avoid these options unless you add unrefined, natural mined salt or sea salt (which contain about 80 natural minerals). Some healthy salt choices include Redmond Salt, Celtic Salt or Himalayan salt. Add a little apple cider vinegar, if desired for taste. Use MRT and listen to your instincts when determining the right salt concentration, since your body may need more or less. Find the mixture that tastes best to you, to help you get the minerals you need and increase your desire for life-giving water.

An additional problem with non-spring, bottled water is that it likely comes from filtered city water, which has its own risks. Consider using glass or PET (polyethylene terephthalate) bottles that are free of phthalates and bisphenol A (BPA) for your water, since most other plastic bottles leach harmful chemicals into the water.

CITY WATER, CHLORINE AND FLUORIDE

Is it possible that something so innocent as the water in your faucet is bad for your health? Well, in a word ... yes. City water is cheap and easy to obtain, but it comes with some serious health consequences. The chlorination process, which kills bacteria in the water, also has some poisonous side-effects. This process creates trihalomethanes, haloacetic acids, bromate and chlorite, which in turn cause bladder and rectal cancer in humans.[52]

The U.S. Council of Environmental Quality determined that the cancer risk for people who drink chlorinated water is nearly twice that of those who drink un-chlorinated water.[53]

> *The behavioral pattern that results from the use of fluoride matches that produced by cancer treatment that causes a reduction in intelligence.*
>
> *– Dr. Phyllis Mullenix*
>
> Dr Phyllis Mullenix: The "Miracle Of Fluoride" or a Dirty Industry?, www.fluoridationfacts. com/education/propaganda/980100_mullenix. htm (January 2014).

Moreover, city water supplied to 41 million Americans is contaminated with prescription drugs, likely from drugs that have been flushed down the toilet.

Years ago, city water departments decided to put fluoride in drinking water because it was thought to strengthen teeth and bones with no negative side effects. We know better now. Research studies have confirmed that fluoride lowers intelligence, makes bones brittle, causes bone cancer, causes brain damage, causes kidney damage and leads to early sexual maturation. What's more, dental studies of more than 39,000 people that spanned over 50 years have shown absolutely no benefits and higher toxicity for those who drink fluoridated water.[54]

Health risks are significant for people who shower using city water, since the body absorbs water and toxic products directly through the skin,

---

52   R.D. Morris et al., *Chlorination, Chlorination By-Products, and Cancer: A Meta-Analysis, American Journal of Public Health*, July 1992, 82(7): 955–963.

53   Sadhna Vora, *There's Something in the Water! A Look at Disinfection By-Products in Drinking Water*, http://legacy.jyi.org/ volumes/volume5/issue4/features/vora.html (January 2014).

54   Heidi Stevenson, *EPA Scientists Oppose Water Fluoridation*, http://healthimpactnews.com/2013/epa-scientists-oppose-water-fluoridation/ (January 2014).

as well as by inhalation. One study revealed nearly double the risk of colon cancer for those who regularly drank, showered, bathed or swam in chlorinated water.[55] You absorb up to six times more harmful chemicals through your lungs and skin while bathing than from simply drinking city water.[56]

Think twice before using city water, especially given the large volume of water that filters through your body each year. If you simply must drink city water, get a high-quality, under-sink or whole-house filter, and don't forget to change the filter regularly. Get a good shower filter for the bathroom. If you don't *have* a filter, *you are the filter.*

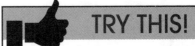

TRY THIS!

MRT: Drinking Water
MRT is explained on page 197.

- *Use MRT while holding glass-bottled samples of spring, reverse osmosis, unfiltered tap, filtered tap and any other drinking water. See which water gives you the best results.*

WATER THERAPY

The skin is the body's largest organ. Many toxins enter the body through your skin since it is not impervious to substances. A seemingly harmless dip in a swimming pool, for example, will likely result in elevated levels of toxic chlorine and bromine in your blood. Chlorine and bromine are both endocrine disruptors which can, in time, precipitate a host of disorders, from thyroid or adrenal dysfunction to cancers. If you have a hot tub or a swimming pool, consider using natural alternatives to chlorine such as baking soda or food-grade hydrogen peroxide. My wife and I converted our hot tub to an ozone purification system. Our swimming pool has a silver and copper ionization system. Australians and Europeans have used natural water plants for swimming pool filtration for many years. If you are regularly in public swimming pools or if you have a child on a school swimming team, consider using homeopathic remedies to neutralize the harmful effects of the toxic chemicals in the water.

Maybe you've heard of the crazy people who jump half-naked into a lake or ocean in the middle of the winter just for fun. I actually believe they

55   Villanueva et al, *Bladder Cancer and Exposure to Water Disinfection By-Products through Ingestion, Bathing, Showering, and Swimming in Pools,* American Journal of Epidemiology, 2007, 165(2): 148–156.

56   *Shower Water Toxicity,* www.pacifichealthcenter.com/blog/?page_id=203 (January 2014).

are not so crazy as you might think. "Capillary isometrics" means alternately stimulating your body with hot and cold water. The effect is to promote healthy circulatory functions. Our distant ancestors never had hot showers, but instead they may have dunked in the lakes and streams all year round.

You practice capillary isometrics when you shower at a reasonably warm temperature, gradually turning the temperature cooler. Repeat several times, finishing with comfortably cool water. See if you don't grow to love it as much as I do. The benefits include more energy, strengthened nervous system, stimulated metabolism, increased adaptability to changing temperature and weather, better blood flow and healthier hair and skin.

Relieve the minor pain of hemorrhoids, anal fissures, bladder infections, irritated prostate, vaginal infections, inflammatory bowel disease, episiotomies and uterine cramps by taking a sitz bath in your bathtub. Simply immerse yourself in tepid water up to your hips. Add Epsom salt, apple cider vinegar or essential oils if desired.

Other refreshing and revitalizing water therapies include taking a dip in natural hot springs, or simply walking barefoot in the rain or on the dewy grass. The chapter on Essential #6: Nature says more about the amazing benefits of grounding yourself to the earth, and grounding has extra benefits whenever water is involved.

Water is the best and most easily accessed medicine on the planet. It is all around us, and yet we often take it for granted. Drink it. Bathe in it. Immerse yourself in it. Receive this priceless, healing, life-giving gift of nature with a thankful heart.

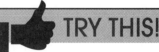

TRY THIS!

MRT and TIP: I Love Water
(see Essential #8 for help using MRT and TIP)

- *Use MRT to test positive statements such as, "I am losing my taste for all unhealthy drinks. I want to be healthy and hydrated. I want to drink more water. I love drinking water. Water is good for me. I am hydrated. I am a water drinker."*
- *Use TIP while repeating weak statements. Retest with MRT.*
- *This technique can be applied to all Eight Essentials.*

Our free, Whole Person Appraisal at www.DrFrankKing.com will help you identify additional ways to plug the holes in your wholeness that are robbing you of life-giving water!

SELF-EVALUATION
WATER

My Life-Destroying Choices (e.g.: too much sugar-based drinks, not enough water, poor quality of water)	**My Life-Affirming Choices** (e.g.: develop a taste for water, listen to my thirst, drink more pure water
1	1
2	2
3	3
4	4
5	5
6	6
7	7

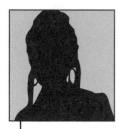

Bella's Story:
The Kitchen Detective

"Hey Daddy. Look at this."

My 12-year-old daughter Bella showed me the backs of her hands. They were covered with a red rash. White scaling cowered in the cracks between her fingers.

"Does it hurt?" I asked.

"No. It's just red and rough."

"It could be a reaction to the cold weather," I said. The January mountain air in Western North Carolina can be brutal. "Keep your hands warm and moist and let's see if that helps."

When that didn't help, I suspected that a food allergy might be causing the eczema on Bella's hands.

"Meet me in the kitchen," I told her. "Let's see if you are allergic to anything you're eating."

Bella has been doing Muscle Response Test (MRT) with me since she was young, so we got straight to business in the kitchen.

She held some wheat bread in one hand while I tested her other arm.

Her muscle was firm as a rock.

I gave her a box of crackers.

She was steady and strong.

I gave her a natural energy bar.

Down her arm went, weak as a willow twig.

"Wow," said Bella. "Do you think that's the problem?"

"Maybe, but let's keep testing," I suggested. "You might only be allergic to some of the ingredients in that bar."

I gave her a dried fruit and oat bar.

She was strong.

I gave her a peanut butter bar.

Down her arm went.

"I think we're getting closer," I said. "Try this."

I gave her a jar of peanut butter.

Down her arm went.

I gave her a can of peanuts.

Down her arm went.

"I think we found it, Dad," she said with big smile on her face.

We read the ingredients in the energy bar and sure enough, peanuts were listed.

From that moment, Bella stopped eating peanut butter, peanuts and peanut ingredients. In a week, the eczema was nearly gone. In two weeks, her hands were free from all traces of rash.

Bella avoids all peanut products and has been rash-free ever since that day, thanks to some thoughtful kitchen detective work.

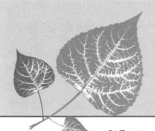

ESSENTIAL #4:
FITNESS

What used to be about burning calories is now more about burning up what is false. Lies I used to tell myself about who I was and what I could do, friendships that cannot withstand hills or miles, the approval I no longer need to seek, and solidarity that cannot bear silence. I run to burn up what I don't need and ignite what I do.

– Kristin Armstrong, "Mile Markers: The 26.2 Most Important Reasons Why Women Run"

When it came to healthy nutrition, Wanda scored 11 ... on a scale of one to ten. She was extremely knowledgeable about supplements and had probably read every book that had ever been written about nutrition.

"But I'm always so tired," she told me. "I have to literally drag myself out of bed in the morning, and I can barely function after being awake for several hours. Now my husband lost his job, and I don't know if I can afford to keep taking all my nutritional supplements."

> *Every human being is the author of his own health or disease.*
>
> **– Hindu teacher and yoga master Sivananda Saraswati**

"Is that so?" I asked. "It sounds like you're taking a lot of pills."

Wanda gulped. "I spend two hundred dollars each week on supplements."

I was aghast. I saw this as confirmation that something was out of whack in her life.

Wanda had a pear-shaped figure and was about 40 pounds overweight. She ate healthy meals but she never exercised. Her eyes, her voice, her whole posture sent signals of fatigue and lethargy.

"I'm such a homebody," she said, slumped down in my office chair. "I love my work, but I sit at my desk most of the day. I don't like getting outside. I hate to sweat or get dirty. That's just not me."

I gave her a doctor's prescription. Lucky for her, this prescription didn't cost much.

"Fresh air and sunshine," was the doctor's orders. "Get outside and get moving. Walk briskly for 20 to 30 minutes a day. Come back in a week and we'll see how you're feeling."

Seven days later Wanda returned. Her face looked brighter and her movements were more animated.

"I'm feeling better already," she said. "And I'm taking less supplements."

After a month of physical activity, she looked and felt terrific. She had quit all but a few nutritional supplements.

"Congratulations," I told her. "You look wonderful, and you have so much more energy."

"I do," Wanda said, "and I don't even know where it comes from. I've lost weight without even trying! My whole outlook on life is more positive. I actually look forward to going on walks. And my husband is thrilled that I'm saving nearly two hundred dollars a week. Did I tell you that I've gotten him to go on walks with me?"

Wanda had changed from a victim to a victor. She had taken back her health simply by adding one more of the Eight Essentials to her routine.

AWKWARD ZOMBIES

Wanda's story illustrates how six or seven essentials are not enough. You might eat, drink, think and sleep well and still be dying inside. Wanda's whole life changed when she learned that her "Declaration of Independence" in the Healing Revolution was a break with her sedentary lifestyle, and a commitment to get more fresh air, sunshine and exercise.

The 21st century lifestyle is turning us into awkward zombies. A zombie moves slow, avoids the sunlight, eats junk, avoids physical activity, is antisocial and has a short existence. Many people walk like uncoordinated zombies, having failed to learn natural cross-crawl motion (to be described later). Many of us are in good shape ... as long as "round" is the right shape. Just kidding.

Sadly, 80 percent of U.S. adults are not getting enough exercise. Only about 20 percent of Americans meet the physical activity recommendations established by the Centers for Disease Control and Prevention. These guidelines include 2 ½ hours per week of moderate aerobic activity such as walking, or 1 ¼ hours of intense aerobic activity such as jogging, in addition to muscle-strengthening activities such as push-ups, sit-ups or weight-lifting.[57]

Studies show that you can *add two years to your life* simply by reducing the time you sit each day to less than three hours. Moreover, you can *add 1.38 years to your life* by watching less than two hours of television per day.[58] Just think of all the terrific things you could do if you were to be given those extra years of healthy, happy life!

Research also shows that short bursts of intense exercise, such as 30-second sprints done three times a week (for a total of only 90 seconds per week), are very beneficial for strengthening the heart and arteries. High-intensity exercise causes the capillaries to dilate, maintaining the arteries' flexibility even into the later years of life.[59] My suggested plan for fitness includes about 10 minutes a week of Peak Fitness Exercises, which are intense sprint-like bursts.

DISCOVER YOUR PASSIONS

Perhaps you desire to become more physically fit. That's great! The challenge, then, is to stick with the program. One disheartening fact I've noticed is that exercise has one of the highest failure rates of all the Essentials in my patient's lives. Why? Because people rush into it too fast, choosing an exercise program that they don't like. Three months later the thrill is gone, and so is their

> *A bear, however hard he tries, grows tubby without exercise.*
>
> *– A.A. Milne,*
> *"Winnie the Pooh"*

---

57   *One in Five Adults Meet Overall Physical Activity Guidelines*, www.cdc.gov/media/releases/2013/p0502-physical-activity.html ; see also Mayo Clinic staff, Exercise Intensity: *Why it Matters, How it's Measured*, www.mayoclinic.com/health/exercise-intensity/SM00113 (January 2014).

58   Katzmarzyk PT, Lee I-M. "Sedentary Behaviour and Life Expectancy in the USA: A Cause-Deleted Life Table Analysis," *British Medical Journal Open*, February 2012, e000828, doi:10.1136.

59   Mark Rakobowchuk et al., *Sprint Interval and Traditional Endurance Training Induce Similar Improvements in Peripheral Arterial Stiffness and Flow-Mediated Dilation in Healthy Humans*, American Journal of Physiology, Regulatory, Integrative and Comparative Physiology, July 2008, 295(1): R236–R242.

exercise program. They never discovered that fitness can be fun. Well, I say that fun is the beginning of FUNctional. Functional health is natural and integrated into a whole-life, holistic approach.

One of the most important keys to success is to learn what you love, and be what you love. If you don't love your workout, you will be inclined to give up. If you don't know what activities you love, that only means you haven't discovered them yet. So many diverse and exciting activities are available in the wild world around us. It's like Wanda: she thought she didn't like walking, but that's because she never seriously gave it a go. Discover what activities you love. Cultivate a love for all Eight Essentials.

Here's a little known fact about fitness: it is addictive, and thankfully it's the kind of habit you will *not* want to kick, once you fit it into the natural strides of your daily life.

In this chapter, I'll show you how to transform your life with simply 20 to 30 minutes of physical activities a day. You don't have to sign up for a membership at the gym, although that's a good choice for some people. Fitness happens when you toss a ball or walk a dog, when you climb stairs, when you ride your bike, or when you park the car a few blocks away from your destination. You can even become more fit by simply taking short, two-minute breaks from your job.

Before we get into some of the fitness techniques that have transformed many of my patient's lives, it is important to establish two basics that are foundational to good health: posture and whole-body breathing.

HOW ARE YOU POSTURED?

Most people are impairing their health with poor posture, and they don't even know it. Poor posture commonly causes fatigue, and it negatively affects bones, muscles, glands and organs. Moreover, posture affects attitudes, emotions, social interactions, productivity and even enthusiasm for life. Good posture enhances whole-body breathing, bringing confidence and a positive self-image.

These are a few simple exercises to encourage good posture. Make these exercises a regular part of your daily routine to enhance good health and keep you standing straight for many years to come.

◆ *To identify your best posture, stand with your feet shoulder-width apart* and stretch your hands high above you. Slowly lower your arms to your side without slumping. Note your posture, and remember how it feels. Stand, walk and sit with this posture. If you feel yourself slumping, imagine a string tugging you up from the top of your head. Repeat this exercise several times daily to reset your optimal posture.

◆ To enhance nerve flow to your arms and hands, stretch your arms high above your head while turning the palms of your hands toward each other. Stretch your fingers to the sides and as far down as you can. Hold this posture for 10 to 15 seconds, feeling the gentle burning sensation in your stretched hands, wrists and arms. Do three repetitions. This is a good exercise to proactively avoid carpal tunnel and brachial neuritis symptoms.

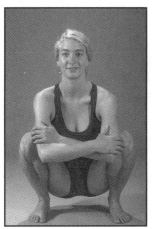

Sitting squat

Squatting is another natural posture that is extremely beneficial for optimum skeletal and internal health. Unfortunately, modern chairs and toilets have robbed us of this healthy position that was common to most cultures throughout history. Squatting creates good balance and strengthens back, pelvis, hips, knees, ankles, feet, digestion and bowels.

◆ *Place your feet shoulder-width apart. Squat down until your thighs are resting on your calves, with your upper arms on or inside your knees. Your feet should be flat on the floor. Simply rest there for 30 to 60 seconds, than rise to a stand. Do three repetitions.*

Stabilize yourself in the squatting position, if necessary for the first few weeks, by holding onto a rope or belt that is securely fastened to a sturdy post or piece of furniture. Additionally, some people find it helpful to put their heels on a short length of 2 by 4 lumber that is lying from side to side, flat on the floor.

Be patient with this exercise, since it may take some time to develop. Once you reset your body to squatting, your internal organs, muscles, tendons and your colon will thank you for many years to come.

WHOLE-BODY BREATHING

Oxygen is what I like to call "vitamin O." Many people suffer from oxygen deficiency, which is linked to chronic illnesses including cancer, respiratory disease, heart disease and a host of other ailments that plague people today. Lack of oxygen is one of the primary causes of fatigue.

This is one of the most easily corrected problems. The cure – vitamin O – is absolutely free for every man, woman and child on the planet. Whole-body breathing heightens energy and alertness. Full diaphragm breathing increases oxygen intake, improves digestive health and improves lymphatic flow. People who breathe deep live longer than shallow breathers. Increased oxygen in the blood stream is believed to decrease bacteria, fungi and even cancer in humans.[60] Shallow breathing is a bad habit that robs many people of life-giving vitamin O.

Full diaphragm breathing happens naturally with aerobic exercise, increasing with the intensity of the workout. Sprinters and long-distance runners don't have to remind themselves to breathe deep; it just happens. People who walk or exercise moderately, on the other hand, might need to be more intentional about practicing deep breathing. People who sit at a desk or in a vehicle most of the day need deep breathing.

The diaphragm is the large muscle between the thoracic and the abdominal cavity. The dropping diaphragm causes the lungs to expand more fully and take in fresh air, while the rising diaphragm forces the spent air out of the lungs. The diaphragm and the heart are the only muscles in your body that never stop moving until your life is over. Therefore, these muscles must remain in excellent health.

To breathe deep, expand your belly, sides and lower back all at the same time. As you do so, your diaphragm will drop to allow the lungs to expand to full capacity. Feel the openness in your throat. Then exhale through your nose, allowing your belly, sides, back and chest to find their natural resting position. Repeat.

Count the seconds it takes you to inhale. Make the exhalation 1 to 2 seconds longer than the inhalation. You may also wish to exhale through your mouth. Practice deep breathing at home, in your car, at school, at work and at all times of the day.

---

60   *Clinical Studies Related to Breathing Development,* www.breathing.com/articles/clinical-studies.htm (January 2014). Optimal Breathing at www.breathing.com has more excellent resources related to deep breathing.

This simple process is the way most people naturally breathe while asleep, but it somehow gets forgotten in the daytime. Many people breathe too shallow, never filling the deeper recesses of the lungs with vitamin O, never fully cleansing the lungs of carbon dioxide and other toxins. You can fight oxygen deficiency when you are sitting, walking or otherwise breathing naturally using your diaphragm.

The lungs are wonderful cleansing mechanisms, so try not to overwhelm them with unhealthy toxins like cigarette smoke. If you do smoke, natural cigarettes are perhaps healthier than regular cigarettes, which contain thousands of ingredients and added chemicals. Still, one full day of cleansing breaths might not be enough to clear your lungs of the pollutants from one inhalation of any kind of smoke. Cigarettes are so addictive that it is best never to start smoking. But don't beat yourself up if you smoke – you are not a bad person! Congratulate yourself for taking small steps in the right direction, like smoking less each day. Use homeopathic remedies and Tap Into Potential (TIP) to help you kick the habit. Deep breathing and natural remedies can help cleanse your body from smoke toxins.

E-cigarettes are becoming quite popular, and preliminary research suggests that they do not have the negative side effects of combustible cigarettes. The vaporizing method used in e-cigarettes might help wean addicted smokers off of nicotine, while not supplying many of the toxic chemicals of cigarettes that burn. They may be a more healthy way to kick the habit and add years to your life.

ENDORPHINS

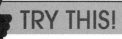 **TRY THIS!**

Yawn... The next time your energy is fading and you're thinking about your standard pick-me-up drink or snack, try spending three minutes on one of the Energizing Techniques explained later in this chapter. The rush of endorphins just might surprise you!

Exercise causes the body to release neurotransmitters called endorphins into your blood stream. Endorphins energize you. They produce a healthy "rush" that is totally natural, totally healthy and infinitely better than any drug you could ever buy on the streets or in a pharmacy. Endorphins give you a whole new positive outlook on life. They sharpen your creativity and awareness, and they make you naturally happy!

If you are emotionally depressed and finding it difficult to be motivated about getting fit, the remedy-times-two is to exercise. Exercise will heal your body while endorphins heal your mind and emotions. Many people measure success in terms of dollars, applause or "likes" on the web; I prefer using endorphins. Endorphins are the feel-good hormones that are free for the taking, and they are just a heartbeat away.

NOW FOR THE EXCUSES ...

Treat yourself like a fat person with aches and pains and a suitcase full of excuses, and good luck – you'll stay exactly where you are. Train like an athlete and, though you may not look like one now, you will become one.

– Chalene Johnson, "PUSH"

Before you rush into anything, stop and ask yourself a few questions. What kind of physical activity do you love to do? Can you sustain this activity all year long, in all kinds of weather? Do you have a back-up rainy-day and snowy-weather activity, like walking at the mall, riding a stationary bike or walking on a treadmill? How will you fit fitness into your daily schedule? How many days per week will you exercise? If all you have are a few minutes during lunch, morning break and afternoon break, that's wonderful. If you have 20 minutes at the beginning or end of the day, three times a week, that's great too. Imagine growing to love this active lifestyle, being happier and healthier for years to come. Your "program" should be manageable, so if in doubt start small, not big. Then give it a try for a few weeks. It generally takes about 20 days to change a bad habit or develop a new healthy habit.

We all face obstacles to staying fit while juggling the competing demands of life in the 21st century. In a typical day, I might drop the kids off at school and then drive a half hour to work where I spend much of the day reading, writing, answering emails, adjusting patients, prescribing remedies or talking on the phone. When I've done my time, I risk my life among the crazy drivers on the freeway. It's a rat race and many people are tempted to buy a greasy burger, grab the television remote and crawl into their caves for a few hours before falling into bed.

You, like me, will encounter a world of reasons why not to exercise: You're too tired or too rushed. It's too cold outside, or too hot, too wet, too dry, too dark, too sunny, too windy, you don't have the right clothes, the dog or child is throwing up, you don't have enough time or you just ran out of peanut butter! Excuses happen, so get them out in the open right here at the start. When I lived in a colder climate, I had objections about exercising in snowy weather. Then I bought a pair of cross-country skis and discovered my hidden passion for that very special winter activity.

> *Exercise is a dirty word. Every time I hear it I wash my mouth out with chocolate.*
>
> *– Cartoonist Charles M. Schulz*

I assure you that there is an answer for every excuse. Some of my most refreshing moments have been when I was so busy I didn't think I had time to exercise, or when I didn't want to walk in the rain or snow. The air is never purer than in the rain or snow, and the appropriate apparel makes these walks not only comfortable, but almost magical. Healthy, happy and well-adjusted people expect the best things in life not to be free and easy. They find ways to get past the excuses. For every excuse, you have an opposing healthy instinct that will lead you to make a life-giving choice. Turn on your healthy instincts.

Most importantly, remind yourself about the positive picture of who you are becoming. Do you desire that awesome picture of a healthy, whole you? Do you believe you can become that person? Never lose track of that beautiful picture of the new you. Use TIP (Tap Into Potential) to reinforce that picture and remind yourself that nobody but you can stop you from being that person. One of my patients said that tapping to the words, "I like exercising," helped her develop a passion for fitness. The secret to success is learning to love it.

Next, find something you like to do – even if it seems small – and just do it. To encourage your progress, you might like to journal or use social media to tell others about your exercise routine. Involve your healing buddies. Tell others about the rewards you are seeing in terms of energy, sleep, body strength, weight loss, mental clarity, emotional health and self-confidence. Get the endorphins flowing. You will be amazed at how the excuses melt away when you are doing what you absolutely love to do.

CROSS-CRAWL AND MIND-BODY COMMUNICATIONS

Another healthy, human function that this modern life of technology, comfort and convenience has robbed from many people is the fundamental, coordinated ability of the brain to communicate with the body.

It goes back to cross-crawl development. Toddlers instinctively practice hetero-lateral movements when they learn to crawl: They move their right hand in sync with their left leg, and vice versa. This creates a healthy communication between brain and body.

Research has shown that some of the devices designed to help toddlers with physical development, including infant walkers and even shoes, in fact interfere with proper development.[61]

Parents give their children a precious gift when they encourage them to play outside, to walk and run on uneven surfaces where they can learn good balance, and to prevent them from spending long hours in an artificially-lit, electronic-device-centered environment. Coordinated mind-body communication is a learned behavior. Kids who sit indoors looking at a screen all day are more likely to become like the awkward zombies I mentioned earlier.

I have seen these uncoordinated zombie kids hurt themselves and constantly spill and break things. My Jewish friend used to call a kid like that a schlemiel; a bungler. They look clumsy when they try to hurry or run, moving homo-laterally, being uncertain of their steps and looking as if they might trip and fall at any time. Coordinated four-year-olds, on the other hand, will skip up and down a steep stairway with a big glass of lemonade in one hand and a guinea pig in the other, singing their favorite song at the top of their lungs.

Natural cross-crawl movement is a sign of healthy brain-body function. Switching is what happens when the healthy functions become confused. On a deeper level, confused signals can lead to serious problems. For example, a stressed liver on the right side of the body may call to the brain for help. The signal goes to the left side of the brain, which prescribes a healing protocol for the liver. That prescription is sent back down to the liver, on the right side

---

61   *True or False: A Baby Who Wears Shoes or Uses an Infant Walker Will Learn to Walk Sooner*, www.wellmont.org/Health-And-Wellness/Health-Library/?eid=156970&lang=1033 (January 2014).

of the body. The brain in a neurologically confused, homo-lateral body may never get the liver's call for help, or it may send help down the wrong side of the body. In my practice, I have often seen people who are suffering from these kinds of switching problems. Whenever someone exhibits homo-lateral tendencies, I frequently find deeper issues with dysfunctional organs or inhibited bodily functions. I have discovered that the majority of people have had at least a minimal level of switching dysfunction.

A sedentary lifestyle with not much exercise and lots of desk-, couch- and car-time may contribute to inhibited brain-body communications. Coordination, balance and memory are inhibited.

Thankfully, switching can be reversed. Your body can learn the cross-crawl functions later in life, even if you missed the first opportunity, although it takes a more intentional approach. Many of the Energizing Techniques (ETs) about to be explained are designed to develop and strengthen cross-crawl functions. Walking and running are some of the most helpful and natural exercises. If you help yourself or someone you know to rediscover hetero-lateral wholeness, you will have brought life to a potential zombie.

> *The American College of Sports Medicine found that the productivity of people after exercise was an average of 65 percent higher than those who did not exercise. If I have something that's really bothering me, so much that it almost hurts my head to try to sort it out, I always find the solution in a puddle of sweat! Intense exercise is like taking a magic pill that gives you the ability to solve problems like a superhero.*
>
> *– Chalene Johnson, "PUSH"*

WHILE AT WORK

An important suggestion for people like me who spend 40 or more hours a week at work or school is to regularly break things up. The last thing you want is to sit at a desk, machine or steering wheel for eight straight hours a day, and then go home and flop on the couch. That kind of activity numbs your mind, inhibits your dexterity and makes you unproductive. It is bad for your brain, muscles, joints, posture, organs, respiration, circulation and lymph flow. It requires intentional whole-body breathing, since sitting can interfere with diaphragm expansion, especially if you slouch.

Over 90 percent of my patients have been affected by lymph congestion. Unlike the circulatory system, the lymph system has no heart-like muscle to pump fluid around. It relies upon bodily motion for circulation. Bodies that are not in motion have stagnant lymphatic systems and are much more susceptible to illness.

I have used an adjustable standing desk with my laptop computer at times. I take short breaks at mid-morning, lunch and mid-afternoon. I like to take short walks down the street with my co-workers, soaking in Doctor Sunshine while sucking in vitamin O.

If necessary, program your computer or cell phone to remind you to take a break. Get up and stretch your arms, legs, neck, head and spine at least once every hour. Get a drink of water and use the bathroom. Breathe deep. Practice Energizing Techniques (ETs) and Two Minute Toning for a mid-day rush that's better than sugar or caffeine. If you snack, eat only healthy vegetables, fruits and whole foods.

I cannot overstate the importance of taking breaks and of regularly exercising. Get those jolly little elves – the happy endorphins – rushing through your body. Ride your bicycle or walk to work. You just might discover a healthy substitute for that mandatory cup of joe.

Try this: spend 10, 20 or 30 minutes exercising before or after work and see if you don't get an hour or two's worth of extra productivity in return. The endorphin euphoria is amazing. Without it, we become workplace zombies, waiting for the Friday afternoon gong that will set us free. You know it's true! At the very least, take a brisk 10 minute walk during lunch or break time and see how wonderful it makes you feel. You'll even save a buck or two that you normally spend on your favorite pick-me-up drink.

THE YOGI MASTER WHO BLEW MY MIND

I crossed paths with another superhero less than a year after I'd been astounded by 80-year-old Paul Bragg, who lectured while standing on his head (page 12). The unassuming man who caught my attention was a yoga practitioner, a martial artist and a master of some of the world's best-kept natural fitness secrets.

This smallish man did not make a positive first impression on me. He looked like a scrawny hippie, sporting a long beard, pony tail, tie-dyed t-shirt, baggy cotton pants, dirty feet and Birkenstock sandals. I vividly recall the moment in his presentation when he held a bucket of water in each hand, his arms held out straight to the side. He held that iron cross position for several minutes.

Then he scanned the auditorium. "Who wants to hold the buckets?"

My hand went up in a flash. The man pointed at me so I eagerly went forward. I was trim, tight and buffed-out from my boxer training. Not only that, but I had carried countless heavy buckets of water to the pigs when I was younger. I hand-watered our livestock at all the fairs we attended throughout the summer months.

If this little guy can do it, then so can I, I thought as I grabbed a bucket in each hand.

My arms went straight out, parallel to the ground.

One ... two ...

As I started counting the seconds, I immediately knew this wasn't going to be easy.

... three ... four ...

I was amazed how quickly the burning started.

... five ...

The pain became intense. Time slowed to a painful crawl.

... six ...

Each second became an eternity. I rushed the count to see if it might help.

... seven-eight-nine ...

My arms started shaking. I was fading fast.

... ten.

I could barely keep the buckets from spilling as they crashed to the floor. My shoulders and arms were in flames. I stared in amazement at the scrawny, little hippie.

How in the world ... ?

I returned to my seat with more of an open mind and a willingness to learn. Next, a massive body builder-type came forward to show us how it should be done. And if anyone could do it, this guy could. His upper arms were thicker than my thighs. His neck was like a pile-driver.

The body builder picked up the buckets and extended his arms. To his dismay, he lasted about the same time as me, crashing and burning in defeat. He headed back to his seat, shaking his head in bewilderment.

"Mr. Yogi" went on to teach me a lesson that I have never forgotten. He explained how conventional exercise and weight training are focused solely on the larger, extrinsic muscles. This man's routine, which included martial arts and several forms of yoga, also developed the intrinsic muscles. He explained the intrinsic energy from the inner chi. Although his biceps were much scrawnier than mine, his inner strength enabled him to hold the buckets of water far longer.

I embraced and developed this man's whole-body approach to exercise. As years passed and my chiropractic, naturopathic career developed, I expanded these techniques and refined them to provide a balance of intrinsic and extrinsic strength training and muscle toning, with range of motion and cross-crawl coordination.

Out of this experience, I developed the Energizing Techniques (ETs). I refined them with my patients, from the flabbiest couch potato to the

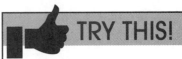

TRY THIS!

MRT and TIP: I Love Fitness

(see Essential #8 for help using MRT and TIP)

- *Use MRT and TIP to attack your greatest obstacles to fitness. For example, say "I have energy to exercise. I have time to exercise. I can enjoy exercising in the dark or rain. I am trading my zombie body for a living, breathing, energetic, hard-working human body!"*

- *Use MRT and TIP while saying "I choose to be physically active. I am a healthy, active person. I love moving my body. Exertion is good for me. I enjoy Energizing Techniques and Strength Training."*

most chiseled Olympian. These ETs have a track record of revitalizing and reenergizing people in all different ages and stages of life. They restore youthful vigor and help prevent injury by energizing the whole body and mind.

That is the story behind the Energizing Technique, and how a yogi master revolutionized my world.

WORK SMARTER, NOT HARDER

Mark Sisson was a fitness monster. He ran over 100 miles a week and earned a qualifying spot for the 1980 U.S. Olympic trials. He finished fourth in the extremely popular Hawaii Ironman Triathlon in 1982. Unfortunately, Mark was forced to stop running due to osteoarthritis, tendonitis and a compromised immune system.

"The inhuman amount of training and weekly racing was taking its toll, and I found myself constantly sick or injured," says Mark. "Unfortunately, the popular wisdom of the past 40 years – that we would all be better off doing 45 minutes to an hour a day of intense aerobic activity – has created a generation of over-trained, under-fit, immune-compromised exerholics."[62]

Too many people choose to not exercise at all, rather than follow the "exerholic" program, not realizing that their health could improve significantly simply by walking as little as 10 minutes a day.

Today, Mark advocates a more thoughtful, moderate approach to exercise. And he is right. You can accomplish much more by working smarter, not harder.

The human body is designed for a lifetime of natural (not repetitive) movement and activity, interspersed with short bursts of intense exercise. The human body's fight or flight mechanism harkens back to more primal times when people unexpectedly faced threats from wild animals or enemies, when they were forced to either fight a brief battle or run a short distance to safety.

For this reason, I do not advise people to practice intense running or killer workouts. My fitness plan embraces a reasonable program of walking, Energizing Techniques for flexibility and range of motion, Two Minute Toning

62   Mark Sisson, www.marksdailyapple.com/about-2/mark-sisson/#axzz2gPMip36Z and *The Case Against Cardio*, www.marksdailyapple.com/case-against-cardio/#ixzz2gUs9xS2T (January 2014).

for strength and muscle tone, and Peak Fitness Exercises for those short bursts of energy.

Here is a practical plan for daily fitness that I have practiced for many years:

◆ *Spend 10 to 20 minutes a day walking or running.*
◆ *Spend 7 to 10 minutes a day on Energizing Techniques.*
◆ *Spend 4 to 8 minutes a day on Two Minute Toning.*
◆ *Spend 15 minutes a week on Peak Fitness Exercises.*
◆ *Rest 1 day a week if desired (but I suspect you will love it too much to stop).*

This is a simple, life-giving fitness routine: about 30 minutes a day. It's not a magic number, though. Start with only a fraction of this routine, if that's all you can manage at first. You'll see positive returns on any investment that you can make. Try it or tweak it for two or three weeks and you'll probably be hooked for life. See if you don't feel much better and grow to love the new you.

WALKING (10 TO 20 MINUTES A DAY)

> *Grandpa started walking three miles a day when he was 60 years old. He's 97 now, and we don't know where he is.*

Walking is perhaps the simplest, most natural form of exercise. I enjoy walking alone, with pets or with people – all have their benefits. I usually wear comfortable shoes, but it feels terrific to walk barefoot in the morning dew. Sometimes I walk with no agenda other than to enjoy the mountain views surrounding our home. Other times I walk on errands, to look over the animals or to check on the fruit trees or fence line. I breathe deep, oxygenating my body, enjoying the elevated level of endorphins dancing through my bloodstream.

Here's an interesting fact: three brisk ten-minute walks a day are as effective at lowering blood pressure as one 30-minute walk.[63] So if all you have are 10 minutes before, after and during work or school, that's perfect. You need not take precious time away from your family or your

---

63   Barbi Lieberman, *The Walking Trick That Lowers Blood Pressure*, www.prevention.com/health/health-concerns/walking-trick-lowers-blood-pressure (January 2014).

evening routine. Still if you'd rather get a membership at the gym and walk on a treadmill several times a week while watching your favorite television program, then do it.

Outdoor walking is always better than walking on a machine, since the uneven surfaces and changing directions of natural walking will engage more muscles and tendons. Repetitive motions on exercise machines lead to stress, strain and repetitive-motion injuries. It is better to exercise on a machine than not at all, but use different machines and different exercises.

If you truly desire a long, healthy life, then walk. It is the most primal, natural human exercise. Swing each arm naturally in synch with the opposite foot, strengthening your cross-crawl functionality and mind-body balance. Break up the repetitive motions of a daily walk by hopping, skipping or walking backwards from time to time. Change things up by riding your bike, jogging or going for a swim. Most importantly, keep an open mind and discover a diversity of activities that you can't help but love for the rest of your life.

ENERGIZING TECHNIQUES (ETS; 7 TO 10 MINUTES A DAY)

If there was only one set of exercises I could do for the rest of my life, I would choose the Energizing Techniques (ETs). These are the most powerful fitness tools in the Healing Revolution. They revitalize and restore physical and mental health by using therapeutic postures, range of motion, breathing, stretching and contracting. They bring balance, coordination, muscle tone and strengthening of muscles, tendons, ligaments and joints, both extrinsically and intrinsically. Moreover, each muscle corresponds to an internal organ by way of acupuncture meridians and neural pathways, so your organ health is also improved by Energizing Techniques.

ETs can be done anytime, anywhere by anyone. I developed and refined these ETs with many patients for nearly 40 years. ETs combine the best elements of applied kinesiology, naturopathic, chiropractic, yoga, tai chi, qigong, shibashi, physical therapy, isometrics, primal postures and a few other tricks I learned from working with my patients.

Energizing Techniques are a great way to boost your energy level and heighten awareness. They are more fulfilling than caffeine or sugar. It is best not to do all the ETs too close to bedtime, because of the rush of adrenaline and energy, although simple muscle stretching can enhance your sleep time.

The KEYS to ET SUCCESS are: 1) the growing intensity of contraction to your maximum ability that increases over time, 2) using your full range of motion, 3) deep whole-body breathing to super-oxygenate your body, 4) developing an intimate awareness and communication with your body, 5) recharging yourself by visualizing energy flowing into your contracting muscles, and 6) practicing ETs daily.

GENERAL INSTRUCTIONS

♦ *Complete three sets of each ET on each side of your body when applicable (alternating left, right, left, right, left, right). Do more than three sets if your body is begging for more. You'll understand what I mean as you do the ETs.*

♦ *Start relaxed, then increase intensity and range of motion throughout each set. If you push yourself, you can actually work up a sweat and get out of breath from these simple ETs.*

♦ ***See your healthcare provider if you have persistent pain. Listen to your body and lighten up if you experience pain.***

♦ *Practice full diaphragm breathing throughout, in synchronization with the cycles of motion. Hold each position for at least one full breath, or about 10 seconds.*

♦ *Try making groans, grunts, shouts and facial grimaces that match the intensity of your effort. The greater your investment, the higher your return of energy and vitality.*

♦ *Going barefooted or sock-footed is helpful for many ETs.*

♦ *In addition to the basic ETs, you can add your own personalized variations. Be creative!*

♦ *You may discover that some muscle rotations or movements are more clumsy or difficult for you to perform than others. Put more effort into these movements until they become natural. This will strengthen your balance and coordination, even into the later years of life.*

♦ *Muscle cramping is often a sign of magnesium deficiency. Natural magnesium supplements can help if you have a problem with cramping.*

♦ *Find videos and more helpful information about ETs at www.DrFrankKing.com.*

TWO POSTURES

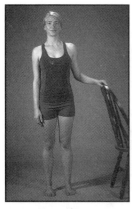

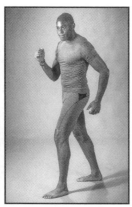

- **Normal Stance:** Stand upright with your feet shoulder-width apart, with one hand holding the wall or furniture for balance.
- **Runner's Stance:** Stand with your feet shoulder-width apart. Step forward with your left foot, bringing your right hand forward and your left hand back, as if you are power

Normal Stance   *Runner's Stance*

walking or sprinting. When it is time to take the alternate posture, skip or step to bring your right foot and left hand forward.

CAUTION: If you have health issues or are at risk of injury, consult with your healthcare practitioner before doing any of these exercises. Never force a motion if you experience pain.

FEET AND ANKLES (NORMAL STANCE)

▶ *Added benefit: This ET enhances bladder health.*

Rotate your ankle clockwise in a wide circular range of motion three times, contracting all the muscles in your foot and ankle, while breathing intensely with your whole body. Lift and expand your toes in the upward circle and curl down in the lower circle. Repeat three times clockwise and three times counterclockwise on each foot, increasing the intensity of contraction and range of motion with each rotation.

Practice intense, whole-body breathing with each ET. Exhale one to two seconds longer than inhaling.

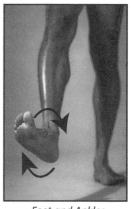

Feet and Ankles

LOWER LEG FLEX
(SHIN AND CALF) (NORMAL STANCE)

▶ *Added benefit: This ET enhances bladder and adrenal gland health.*

Bring your foot forward and point your toes upward in full range of motion, tightening the muscles in your shin (the front of your lower leg). Next bend your knee, contract your calf muscles and extend your foot back as far as you comfortably can. Repeat three times on each leg.

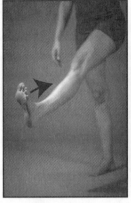 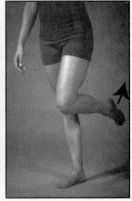

Lower Leg: Shin   *Lower Leg: Calf*

UPPER LEG
(QUADRICEPS AND HAMSTRINGS) (NORMAL STANCE)

▶ *Added benefit: This ET enhances kidney, intestine and adrenal gland health.*

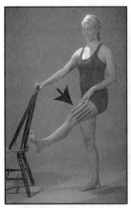 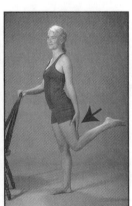

Upper Leg: Quadriceps   *Upper Leg: Hamstring*

Bring your foot forward, locking the knee while tightening the quadriceps muscles in the front of your thigh, feeling the contraction with your hand. Next extend your foot backwards up to your buttocks with bent knee, while tightening the hamstring muscle in the back of your thigh. Use your hand to feel the hamstring muscle tighten in the back of your upper leg. (If you don't feel much tightness now, don't be discouraged – you soon will as you practice ETs.) Do three sets, alternating sides.

Several of these ETs appear to be similar to each other, but you will actually be isolating unique muscle groups in each ET.

BUTTOCKS
(RUNNER'S STANCE WITH LEFT FOOT FORWARD)

▶ *Added benefit: This ET enhances reproductive health.*

Contract your right buttock muscle. Reach back with your left hand and feel the tightness of your buttocks muscle. Hold for about 10 seconds while deeply breathing in and out. Switch your stance to contract the left buttocks. Do three sets, alternating sides.

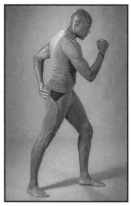

Buttocks

ABDOMINALS
(RUNNER'S STANCE WITH LEFT FOOT FORWARD)

▶ *Added benefit: This ET enhances digestion and small intestine health.*

Contract your left stomach muscles while tilting the upper half of your body slightly forward. Use your right hand to feel your left stomach muscles tighten. Hold for about 10 seconds while deeply breathing in and out. Switch your stance to contract the right stomach muscles. Do three sets, alternating sides.

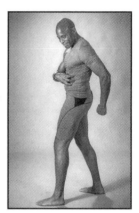

Abdominals

OBLIQUE ABDOMINALS
(RUNNER'S STANCE WITH LEFT FOOT FORWARD)

▶ *Added benefit: This ET enhances digestion and small intestine health.*

Fully twist your trunk to the left and extend your left arm behind you, tilting your body slightly forward. Contract the muscles in your left side. Hold for about 10 seconds while deeply breathing in and out. Switch your stance to contract the muscles on your right side. Do three sets, alternating sides.

Increase the intensity with each ET repetition.

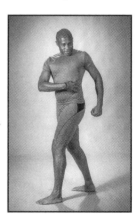

Oblique Abdominals

DIAPHRAM
(NORMAL STANCE)

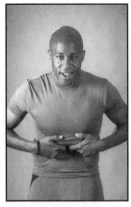
Diaphram

▶ *Added benefit: This ET enhances digestive health.*

Surprisingly, most adults do not breathe properly. Inadequate oxygen intake contributes to poor health. This ET helps you to use your trunk to fill your entire lungs. It exercises your internal organs and glands.

Place your open hands on your belly and breathe in, pushing your hands out as far as you can with your expanding belly. Stand proud and tall but do not raise your shoulders. Feel your belly, sides, back and throat expand as you inhale. Exhale slowly (8 to 10 seconds) while drawing your belly back toward your spine as far as you can. Repeat three times.

As you become comfortable with this ET, exaggerate all movements, inhaling and exhaling to maximum capacity for the benefit of your internal organs and glands.

As you become more comfortable, try improvising and making up your own variations. ETs are even more effective when performed in different ways.

REPRODUCTIVE ORGANS
(NORMAL STANCE)

▶ *Added benefit: This ET enhances circulation and reproductive health.*

Tighten the pelvic floor (kegel) muscles in your lower groin and genitals, as if interrupting urination. Hold while breathing in slowly to full capacity. Then exhale slowly, releasing your muscle contractions. Repeat three times.

UPPER CHEST AND BACK
(RUNNER'S STANCE WITH LEFT FOOT FORWARD)

▶ *Added benefit: This ET enhances liver and stomach health (chest muscles), spleen health (upper-back muscles), thyroid, pancreas and heart health (mid-back muscles), and large intestine, appendix and urinary tract health (lower-back muscles).*

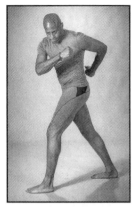

Chest and Back

Contract the right pectoral muscles in your chest, while drawing your right elbow across your abdomen to the left and extending your left arm behind you. Simultaneously contract the left muscles in your back, optionally using your left hand to feel your back muscles tighten. Hold for about 10 seconds while deeply breathing in and out, feeling an intense contraction in your entire trunk. Switch your stance to contract the left muscles in your chest and the right muscles in your back. Do three sets, alternating sides.

SHOULDERS
(NORMAL STANCE)

▶ *Added benefit: This ET enhances lung health.*

Inhale deeply as you raise your hands up from your sides, bending your elbows and bringing your fists over and across the top of your head, while contracting your shoulder deltoid muscles and the upper-trapezius muscles between your neck and shoulders. Then exhale as you slowly bring your arms down in front of you, coming to rest around your chest in a hugging position, keeping your shoulder muscles tightly contracted. Relax and drop your arms to your side. Repeat three times.

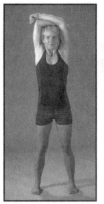
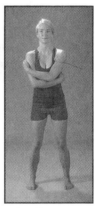

Shoulders Up   *Shoulders Down*

Try improvising, like contracting your shoulder muscles while rotating your arms backward in a circular motion.

Feel free to do more than three sets of each ET for greater results.

UPPER ARMS
(RUNNER'S STANCE WITH LEFT FOOT FORWARD)

▶ *Added benefit: This ET enhances stomach health (biceps) and pancreas health (triceps).*

Bend your right arm and point your right elbow up and in front of you, tightening the biceps muscles in your upper arm. Extend your left arm straight back while contracting the triceps muscles in the back of your upper arm. Raise both arms as high as you comfortably can while contracting your muscles. Relax. Do three sets, alternating sides.

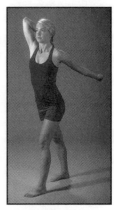

Upper Arms

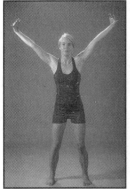

Lower Arms, Hands, Wrists

LOWER ARMS, HANDS AND WRISTS
(NORMAL STANCE)

▶ *Added benefit: This ET enhances stomach health.*

Raise your straightened arms to your side at a 45 degree angle stretched toward the sky, palms facing forward. Open and close your fingers to the extreme while rotating your hands in a circle. Repeat while rotating in the opposite direction. Repeat three times.

FRONT AND SIDE OF NECK
(RUNNER'S STANCE WITH LEFT FOOT FORWARD)

▶ *Added benefit: This ET enhances sinus health.*

Contract your front-left neck muscles while looking to the left. Inhale deeply, feeling your neck muscles with your right hand. Then exhale and straighten your head, relaxing your muscles. Switch your stance and contract your front-right neck muscles. Do three sets, alternating sides.

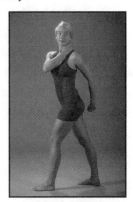

Front of Neck

BACK OF NECK
(NORMAL STANCE)

▶ *Added benefit: This ET enhances sinus health.*

Tilt your face up while tightening the muscles in the back of your neck. Then return your head to the upright position. Repeat three times.

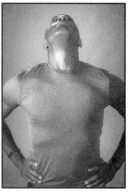

Back of Neck

NECK ROLL
(RUNNER'S STANCE WITH LEFT FOOT FORWARD)

▶ *Added benefit: This ET enhances sinus health.*

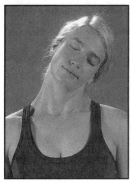

Neck Roll

Tilt your head to the front-left, then rotate it back and to the left, intensely contracting your muscles through the full range of motion, completing three-quarters of a counter-clockwise rotation. Switch your stance and roll your head in the opposite direction. Repeat three times, alternating sides. Many people will experience a pleasant popping sound, providing the added benefit of aligning the neck vertebrae.

FACE
(NORMAL STANCE)

Inhale while yawning dramatically, exaggerating the movements of jaw, mouth, cheeks, eyes, ears, nose, forehead and neck, while contracting all the muscles of your face, head and jaw. Make faces! Yawning replenishes oxygen, relieves facial stress and enhances cerebral spinal fluid in your brain, bringing greater clarity and creativity. Relax after exhaling,

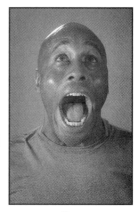

Face

then perform the opposite of a yawn by squeezing your face together like a wrinkled prune. Repeat three times.

Firmly contract your cheek muscles for as long as you comfortably can, and notice the improvement in your smile!

FORTY WINKS
(NORMAL STANCE)

Wink one eye twenty times, expanding and contracting the orbital muscles around your eye to the extremes. Do two sets, alternating sides for a total of forty winks per side. Are you feeling sleepy yet? Probably not, with the extra charge of energy that these ETs will give you.

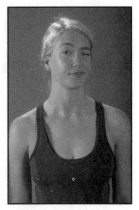

Winks

BRING IT ALL TOGETHER
(RUNNER'S STANCE WITH LEFT FOOT FORWARD)

I like to finish with a big ending that brings all the Energizing Techniques together in one routine. In the Runner's Stance, contract all the muscles in the front of your lower-left body as well as the back of your upper-right body. Hold for about 10 seconds while deeply breathing in and out. Switch your stance to contract the front, lower-right body and back, upper-left body muscles. Repeat three times. Be creative, adding your hand, face and neck muscles. With practice, you will contract nearly every muscle in your body. This full-body ET is so intense that you should be breathing hard to catch your breath by the time you finish.

Congratulations! You have intensely reset and synchronized your whole body and mind. Your vitality has been renewed, released, rewired, restored and recharged. Your flabbiness is turning to firmness. Now enjoy the heightened sense of energy, strength and alertness.

▶ *Videos and helpful articles about Fitness are available at www.DrFrankKing.com.*

Dry Brush Massage

Massage your body, head and limbs using a natural bristle, long-handled body brush with a detachable head, to enhance skin health, increase lymph drainage and prevent tissue sludge. Concentrate on areas that are begging for attention, as well as on fatty areas where you'd like to lose a weight.

Dry brush massage is a natural, effective way to beautify sagging skin. Not one of my patients who lost over 100 pounds needed the needless and expensive skin reduction surgery that so many doctors recommend. Instead, they faithfully dry-brushed their skin, which stimulated it to shrink naturally to its healthy size while actually aiding in the weight-loss process by helping the fatty tissue to disperse.

Listen to your body. What is it telling you? Most likely, your body will be saying, "Ahh ... That's nice. I feel better now. I feel more life radiating from within me. I have more vitality and energy. I feel as if I'm ready to sprint a quarter mile!"

Your body may be begging for more attention in specific areas. If so, give it what it wants. Do more than three sets of exercises in areas that are weak or lacking in full range of motion. ET revitalizes your muscles, glands and organs, awakening your full mind and body potential. It develops both internal and external strengths, as the yogi master taught me. It raises your quality of life to a higher level. It works transcendently to integrate your health and wholeness. Expect exciting things to happen as you set off on this ET journey.

TWO MINUTE TONING
(STRENGTH TRAINING; 4 TO 8 MINUTES A DAY)

ETs are important for overall health. They help restore muscle and joint coordination, balance, memory, clarity of thought and more. Strength training is important for adding strength and muscle tone. As bodies age, muscle mass tends to be lost and is often replaced with fat. The sedentary person drops a six pack and begins to carry a keg around the waist.

The best recommendation is to practice both Two Minute Toning and ETs to build and maintain maximum physical strength and flexibility, while energizing and bringing emotional stability. Fabulous results are gained through a small investment in time and energy.

DR. KING'S TWO MINUTE TONING

Each strength training routine takes about two minutes. Choose two or more of these routines to do each day. Do them during TV commercials, while waiting for friends or family, or when you make a pit stop during a long drive. Like ETs, they are perfect for filling the time cracks in your day, so you can never say you are too busy to stay fit. It's amazing to feel and experience the dramatic results you can get from simply moving. Like a stagnant pond, the inactive body accumulates toxic fluids and grows nasty things. The inner zombie starts to suck the life out of you. All you have to do is shake your bootie a little, do the Hokey Pokey and turn yourself around a little in order to feel and look like a million bucks.

As with ETs, increase intensity with each Two Minute Toning repetition. Feel the muscles burn. Breathe deeply. Grunt, groan and shout if you like. Improvise and add your own twists to the routines. Don't perform Two Minute Toning within a couple hours of bedtime or you may have trouble getting to sleep. Do not push yourself too hard or too fast and risk injury.

CAUTION: If you have health issues or are at risk of injury, consult with your healthcare practitioner before doing any of these exercises. Never force a motion if you experience pain.

SQUATTING EXERCISE

Place your feet shoulder-width apart. Squat down: not all the way, but to where your thighs are parallel with the floor. Rise halfway while tensing your thighs, but do not straighten your legs. Repeat 10 to 15 times (one set). Take a half-minute break, walking casually and stretching your legs. Do three sets in less than two minutes.

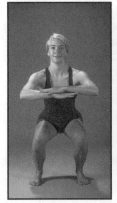
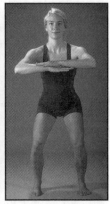

Your range of motion should not take you all the way up or all the way down during this exercise, in order to maintain tension on the upper leg muscle (quadriceps). For a variation as your legs get stronger, hop into the air when rising.

Squat Exercise: Down   *Squat Exercise: Up*

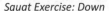

CALF STRETCH AND LIFTS

Stand with the balls of your feet on a stair and your heels hanging off the edge. Hold the handrail for balance. Rise up as high as you can on your tiptoes, then lower your heels as far down as you can. Repeat 30 to 50 times (one set). You will feel a positive burning sensation in your calves. Take a half-minute break. Do three sets in about three minutes.

For an advanced version of this exercise, pull up against the handrail to create more resistance, or hold a heavy weight in your hand.

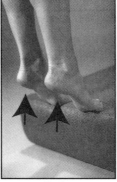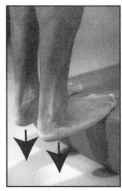

Calf Lifts: Up   *Calf Lifts: Down*

This simple exercise is a good remedy for fatigue, since the calves are linked by meridians to the adrenal glands. Try it the next time you are reaching for a cup of coffee, an energy drink or your favorite pick-me-up, but not before bedtime since the boost in energy is likely to keep you awake for some time.

PUSH-UPS

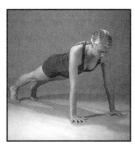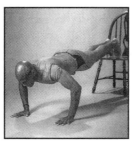

Push-Ups   *Push-Ups: Advanced*

Note: You may want to use push-up handles or two dumbbells if you experience pain in your wrists from doing flat-handed push-ups on the floor.

Place your hands shoulder-width on the floor. Straighten your body with your toes on the floor, while tucking in your belly and chin. Bend your arms at the elbow until your chest and chin barely touch the floor. Push your body back up. Repeat 5, 10 or more times. Take a half-minute break. Work up to three sets of 10 to 30 push-ups in about two minutes. Beginners can place their knees on the floor; experts can place their feet on a chair.

HANGING OUT

Use a pull-up bar for these two exercises. Alternately, you may swing on a sturdy tree limb or hang on monkey bars at the park!

Vertebrae discs shrink and people become shorter with age. This exercise counteracts aging and gravity by opening up joints, circulation and nerve pathways.

Hang by your hands from the bar, lifting your feet off the ground. Hang 30 seconds, or as long as you comfortably can. Take a 10-second break. Do three times in about two minutes. Alternately, lift your knees up toward your chest to strengthen your lower abdominal muscles.

PULL-UPS

Hang with your hands about shoulder-width apart and pull yourself up until the base of your neck touches the bar. Let yourself down slowly. Do three sets of as many pull-ups as you can in about two minutes. Don't be discouraged if at first you aren't good at pull-ups. Build up your strength over time; the rewards will be well worth the effort.

Two Minute Toning is fun, which is the first word in FUNctional. Fight the zombie within. Discover the revitalized, reenergized YOU that you have always hoped to become. You will look and feel a million times better than a zombie! Receive maximum rewards from this simple two minute investment, whenever, wherever you can fit it into your day.

PEAK FITNESS EXERCISES (15 MINUTES A WEEK)

Peak Fitness Exercises involve working up to eight 30-second workout blasts. They get your heart beating in a short amount of time. Peak Fitness stimulates your glandular system in a way that less-extreme exercises cannot. It raises testosterone to an appropriate level for both men and women. It stimulates production of the anti-aging human growth hormone (HGH) which is essential for healing and cell regeneration. Increase HGH production and stay young with Peak Fitness Exercises.

Beginners and people who are out of shape should start with walking or a slower version of this exercise, working slowly up to one short blast. Gradually add more blasts and add higher intensity. Your body will tell you if you are working too hard. When you are fit, your heart will beat hard and your muscles will be tired, but you will feel great.

CAUTION: If you have health issues or are at risk of injuries, consult with your healthcare practitioner before doing any of these exercises. Never force a motion if you experience pain.

Peak Fitness Exercises may be done on a bicycle, recumbent bike, treadmill, elliptical machine or while running. Here is the Peak Fitness program you can follow when you are in good shape:

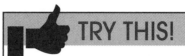 TRY THIS!

TIP: Learning to Love Fitness
(see page 201 for help using TIP)

- *Use Tap Into Potential (TIP) to learn to love fitness.*
- *Tap to statements like, "I love ETs. I love fitness training. I love the new 'me' I am becoming. I am removing all obstacles and excuses to fitness. I am learning to love life and health in all its fullness. This is the new, healthy, beautiful me!"*
- *When excuses come and obstacles to your fitness begin to rear their ugly heads, stop them immediately by using Tap Into Potential. Replace negative thoughts, words and images with positive ones.*

- *Warm up for two or more minutes by walking, jogging or peddling slowly.*
- *Next sprint as hard and as fast as you can for about 30 seconds. SUGGESTION: Try counting breaths instead of seconds; e.g., 20 breaths may equal 30 seconds. You will know you've pushed yourself hard enough if, when you stop, you can NOT say, "Mary had a little lamb" out loud without stopping.*
- *Warm down for about 90 seconds while casually walking or peddling. SUGGESTION: Count breaths instead of seconds; e.g., 33 breaths may be about 90 seconds. The time need not be exact. Some days you might go shorter; other days you will go longer.*
- *Repeat until you have completed eight cycles, or as many as you are comfortable with.*
- *Do Peak Fitness Exercises only once or twice a week.*

Don't push yourself harder than you safely can. For some people, the perfect Peak Fitness Exercise is walking up a steep hill ... or a not-so-steep hill! Gradually work up to the program that feels right for you over the course of several weeks or months.

TAKE BACK YOUR FITNESS
BY LEARNING TO LOVE IT

The fitness plan outlined in this chapter is thoughtfully designed to give you maximum results from a minimum investment of time and effort. Work smarter, not harder. Thirty minutes a day is a good goal for fitness in the Healing Revolution, but if all you have is 30 minutes a week, then take it. If you are like many of my patients through the years, soon you will be taking long walks or bike rides for the sheer fun of it. You will discover an hour or two a week that you didn't even know you had for moving in ways you didn't know you could. Then you will LIVE it by learning to LOVE it!

The tips I've shared in this chapter are effective for helping to minimize many of the chronic problems that plague people today. Our Whole Person Appraisal at www.DrFrankKing.com can help you make more life-affirming choices in all Eight Essentials of life. You'll also find fitness videos and more helpful information about the Healing Revolution at that website. Break out of the zombie crypt. Life is too short to live each day without vitality and strength. Take back your fitness.

SELF-EVALUATION
FITNESS

My Life-Destroying Choices
(e.g.: too little exercise, too many
excuses, fear of working out
in front of others)

My Life-Affirming Choices
(e.g.: develop a life-long passion for
fitness, park farther away from school
or work so I can walk)

My Life-Destroying Choices	My Life-Affirming Choices
1	1
2	2
3	3
4	4
5	5
6	6
7	7

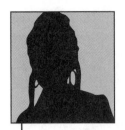

Carol's Story:
Beauty Revived

Carol walked into our health clinic complaining of chronic hip pain. She was about 35 years old with dirty blond hair. She was attractive and had undoubtedly turned a few heads in high school, although now she was 30 to 40 pounds overweight. She had three kids and a husband who worked long hours in construction.

Carol's Whole Person Appraisal was typical of many other people I've seen at her age. Beyond her hip problem, she was fatigued, lethargic, depressed and she had no enthusiasm for her marriage. She was especially frustrated that she couldn't keep her weight down. As for lifestyle habits, she didn't exercise much, she loved sweets and she had a reputation for making outstanding cookies, cakes and baked goods.

Encouraged by the relief she experienced from chiropractic adjustments in the first couple visits, Carol began to share more of her concerns with me.

"I can't seem to get my energy and enthusiasm up these days, Dr. King," she confessed. "I know it sounds silly, but I wish I felt like I did when I was younger." She laughed. "Of course I was a lot thinner then."

"Is that something you would like to work on?" I asked. "Your excess weight may be linked to deeper issues, more than just your hip."

"Sure, I'd lose some weight if I could. But I've tried every diet out there, Dr. King. I spent a lot of money on weight loss products. I starve to death just to lose one pound, then I get it back just *looking* at a donut. Honestly, Dr. King, I don't have much faith in diets anymore."

I laughed. "Neither do I, Carol. But don't worry. My recommendations will not be difficult. Here's something that you can use to get started."

She looked a little surprised when I reached into my bag and pulled out a regular oral thermometer. I told her to take her temperature deep in her armpit each morning. Then I arranged to see her again in a few days.

Carol followed my instructions and brought me the requested temperature readings. We also performed the Ragland's blood pressure test (explained in the HOT Chapter). After putting all the data together, the results were conclusive.

"Your thyroid is shutting down because of high blood sugar, Carol," I explained. "That leads to weight gain, which in turn negatively affects your hip. The blood pressure tests show adrenal fatigue, which causes weakness in your tendons and ligaments. The main contributing factors are first of all, chlorine and fluoride in the city water you drink, and second, the bromine contained in the refined flour and baked goods that you eat. Stress is also a common cause of adrenal fatigue."

"That sounds complicated," she said.

"It's not," I assured her. "I simply recommend that you drink well or spring water, reduce your sugar consumption and eat less white, refined flour. Give it a try for a week or so, then let's see how you're feeling."

Carol eagerly accepted my recommendations. Meanwhile, I helped her find some other healthy, delicious food choices and showed her how a healthy diet (or "live-it," as I like to say) does not mean starving. She replaced refined salt with sea salt and a natural iodine supplement. When she told me she liked to regularly soak in a hot tub, I warned her about the toxic levels of bromine she was absorbing from the dissolved chemicals. She immediately found a more natural alternative to bromine.

Carol began to lose weight, and I had her dry brush-massage her dimply arms, legs and mid-section twice a day (as explained in the Fitness chapter), to restore healthy circulation to her skin.

We did Muscle Response Test and Tap Into Potential to guide her in making healthy lifestyle choices. I gave her a couple of very simple stretching exercises that would fit naturally into the flow of her day. She found more energy and a greater desire for fitness by doing ET exercises, and by joining other walkers in her neighborhood.

Carol's revival was dramatic. Like 80 percent of my patients, she experienced so much more than just the elimination of the one symptom that had driven her to reluctantly pick up the phone and give our clinic a call.

Carol's beautiful arms, legs and face were no longer buried under cellulite. Her energy and enthusiasm for life blossomed. Her marriage even improved. She became a missionary for natural foods and health, bringing her husband, kids and friends into the clinic for help with their issues. She dropped a heavy load from her heart, and the physical results blossomed all around her.

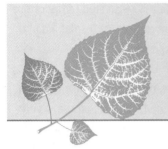

ESSENTIAL #5:
SLEEP

*Blessings light on him that first invented sleep!
It covers a man all over, thoughts and all, like
a cloak; it is meat for the hungry, drink for the
thirsty, heat for the cold, and cold for the hot.
It is the current coin that purchases all the
pleasures of the world cheap, and the balance
that sets the king and the shepherd, the fool and
the wise man, even.*

– Miguel de Cervantes

My son Nathan crawled into my wife's car after school one day, looking pale and fatigued.

"What's the matter, honey?" my wife asked, putting her hand to his forehead. "How do you feel?"

"I feel like crap."

"You're cold and clammy," she said. "Where does it hurt?"

Nathan responded with primal grunts, groans and a few syllables that sounded faintly like "stomach" and "head."

They drove straight home.

"Can I get you some soup," my wife offered, "or a few crackers? You should drink some water."

He refused all offers of help. "I'm going to bed," is all he said as he stumbled up the stairs.

That was mid-afternoon on a Tuesday.

Nathan didn't crawl out of his cave until 7 o'clock the next morning. He'd slept for about 15 hours and when he woke up, he said he felt just fine. Wednesday was business as usual for Nathan, with the pedal to the metal from start to finish.

Other people struggled with that same bug that was going around for maybe a week, never giving their body a chance to heal. But Nathan always does the same thing when he feels sick. He goes into hiber-Nathan ... er, I mean hibernation!

That's always been my first response as well, to sleep when I start feeling sick. Something deep down in the human genes understands the power of sleep to heal.

REST IS THE FIRST PART OF RESTORATION

The amount of sleep required by the average person is five minutes more.

– American playwright Wilson Mizner

Sleep is such a unique and amazing part of life. It brings healing and restoration. Poor sleep is a sure sign that something is out of alignment in one or more of the Eight Essentials. Sleep disturbances are like flashing signals on the instrument panel of life, indicating that one or more of the other Essentials are out of balance. Thankfully the causes of bad sleep are not difficult to identify or fix.

You will spend one third of your life in a revitalizing, repairing, restoring and rejuvenating unconscious state called sleep. Sleep is when your body integrates all Eight Essentials for synergistic healing. People deprived of sleep for extended periods of time have literally gone crazy and died. Inadequate sleep contributes to many disorders including adrenal fatigue, high blood pressure, heart attack, anxiety, depression and more. Insufficient sleep can cut your quality of life in half. A well-rested person is happier, healthier and much more productive.

The quality of sleep is more important than the quantity of sleep. You can regularly sleep eight or nine hours and still be sleep-deprived if you are consistently awakened in the wrong part of your sleep cycle. Eight hours of sleep is a good target figure, but it's not a magic number. Some people need fewer hours because they know how to find that deep, healing sleep.

Everybody can sleep well. You can sleep well, but not because of a magic pill. Natural sleep is one fulfilling, integrated Essential of the Healing Revolution.

STAGES OF SLEEP

These are the natural stages of sleep:

▶ **Stage 1.** This is a relaxed, transitional period between wakefulness and sleep. If awakened from this stage, you will likely say you were not asleep. The average person spends about 7 minutes in this stage of falling asleep.

> *A well spent day brings happy sleep.*
>
> *– Leonardo da Vinci*

▶ **Stage 2.** This stage lasts about 20 minutes, as you lose awareness of surroundings and become perfectly still. The brain begins to produce bursts of fast, rhythmic activity. The body temperature drops.

▶ **Stage 3.** This is a short transitional stage between light sleep and deep sleep. Heart rate, breathing and brain activity all begin to slow down.

▶ **Stage 4.** This is deep, dreamless sleep with the slowest brain activity. Blood pressure, heart rate and breathing rate are all low and stable. Sleepwalking and bed-wetting typically happen at the end of this stage, which lasts up to 30 minutes. You may feel numb and desensitized for up to an hour if awakened from this stage. Eighty percent of human growth hormone, which promotes youthfulness and healing, is released during this stage of sleep. The immune system is strengthened and healed during Stage 4.

▶ **Stage 5.** This stage is called rapid eye movement (REM) sleep because the eyes dart quickly back and forth. This is when dreaming occurs, typically about 90 minutes after you first fall asleep. Respiration and heart rates increase. Brain waves are more active. Body muscles are paralyzed, which is the body's way of preventing you from hurting yourself by actually enacting the physical movements of your dreams. The first nightly REM sleep lasts only a few minutes, then you will awaken or return to Stage 1. You stay in REM sleep longer each time you return, up to about 30 minutes during your final sleep cycle.

In a healthy, restful night, you will cycle through these stages three to four times. The last two stages of sleep are especially essential for good health: Stage 4 restores and heals the body, while Stage 5 REM sleep restores and heals the mind. This is why the quality of sleep is more important than the quantity, although only you can determine the quantity you need to achieve the best quality. These days I sleep nearly nine hours a night, which is longer than I did in past years, and I feel more alert and productive than ever.

INSOMNIA

Few people are actually sleeping to their full potential. Nearly half of all Americans report occasional insomnia, while 22 percent have trouble sleeping nearly every night. The Centers for Disease Control and Prevention calls sleep deprivation a "public health epidemic." People with insomnia are more likely to suffer from avoidable chronic diseases such as hypertension, diabetes, depression, obesity and heart disease. People who have trouble sleeping are four times more likely to suffer from depression than those who sleep well. They miss work more often and receive fewer job promotions.[64]

Insomnia has many causes including stress, anxiety, lack of exercise, stimulants (e.g., caffeine or nicotine), hormonal changes (e.g., menopause), depression, post-traumatic stress disorder and substance abuse. Each one of these problems has a natural, healthy remedy. You could try to throw a sleeping pill at the symptom, but you'd be ignoring the real problem ... while adding more serious risks that are associated with sleeping aids. Natural is better – it's a principle to live by.

I have no objections to taking a half-hour power nap during the day, if that's your way of making up the deficit after a sleepless night. You'll be in good company with people like John F. Kennedy, Winston Churchill, Ronald Reagan, Napoleon, Albert Einstein and Thomas Edison, not to mention many of the longest-living people on earth. A NASA study found that a 40-minute nap improved astronaut performance by 34 percent and alertness by 100 percent.[65] Don't nap longer than 30 or 40 minutes, however, or it might take a long time to recover your alertness and it may make it difficult for you to fall asleep at night. Still, if you are napping because of poor nighttime sleep, it's better to correct the causes of insomnia and "power sleep" all night long.

---

64 *Sleep Aids and Insomnia*, www.sleepfoundation.org/article/sleep-related-problems/sleep-aids-and-insomnia (January 2014).
65 *Napping*, www.sleepfoundation.org/article/sleep-topics/napping (January 2014).

One major cause of insomnia today is the exposure of LED lights from computers, tablets, iPads, iPhones and televisions. A recent study in the journal Applied Ergonomics revealed that viewing self-luminous displays within two hours of bedtime significantly impairs melatonin production, which in turn causes insomnia.[66]

SLEEP DEPRIVATION AND WEIGHT GAIN

> *A good laugh and a long sleep are the best cures in the doctor's book.*
>
> **— Irish Proverb**

The appetite-suppressing hormone leptin and the hunger-triggering hormone ghrelin are largely regulated by sleep patterns. Research shows that people who sleep too little have a significant reduction in leptin levels and an increase in ghrelin, leading to greater hunger and weight gain.[67] Moreover, overweight people are more likely to experience sleep disruptions due to apnea and snoring, contributing to poor sleep quality. It's a vicious circle, reinforced by the depression and feelings of helplessness accompanied by being perpetually tired.

If that's not bad enough, sleep deprivation raises insulin levels, causing further weight gain and increased risk of diabetes. Finally, sleep disturbances cause hormone imbalances that contribute to accelerated aging and decreased mental function.

If you struggle with chronic insomnia or sleep deprivation, remind yourself that you are not just tired: you are sick. Thankfully this is a problem that can be fixed.

Sleep more, have more energy, lose weight and feel great!

MELATONIN

The human body needs melatonin, which can only be produced by the body's pineal gland in absolute darkness.[68] Melatonin makes you sleepy, it slows the aging process and it stabilizes the body's biorhythms. When your

---

66   Wood B, et al, "Light level and duration of exposure determine the impact of self-luminous tablets on melatonin suppression," *Applied Ergonomics*, March 2013, vol. 44, no. 2, 237-240.

67   *Waking Up to Sleep's Role in Weight Control*, www.hsph.harvard.edu/obesity-prevention-source/obesity-causes/sleep-and-obesity (January 2014).

68   See Essential #5: Sleep, for more discussion about the importance of sleeping in a completely dark room.

eyes sense light, your body produces serotonin for greater alertness and it suppresses melatonin production.

Any kind of light hinders melatonin production, but researchers have discovered that LED (light-emitting diodes) displays – and especially blue light wavelengths – are particularly problematic. Blue light occurs in fluorescent light bulbs, cell phones, computers, televisions and devices with LEDs. The closer to bedtime the exposure is, the greater the negative impact upon melatonin production and sleep. A Swiss study showed a dramatic decrease in melatonin production in people who sat in front of computer screens before bedtime. Mental alertness and activity increased, and restful sleep decreased. Insufficient melatonin is also linked to premature aging.[69]

All electronic devices viewed before bedtime are detrimental to sleep, although tablet-style devices are worse because they are typically held closer to the eyes. Studies show that bedtime viewing of electronic devices over the course of several years can contribute to all the more serious risks of sleep deprivation.[70] Another study revealed a 40 percent decrease in melatonin production in people with long exposure to fluorescent lights, compared with those who were exposed to incandescent bulbs.[71]

People experiencing more nighttime light have an increased risk of breast cancer, cardiovascular disease and depression. People who work night-shift jobs are especially susceptible to these harms. Other studies show a correlation between artificial light and obesity, diabetes and sleep disruption.[72]

Even small amounts of nighttime light hinder melatonin production. The light filtering through your closed eyelids may be enough to disrupt your sleep. Install blinds and block out exterior lights entering your room. It is interesting to note that researchers have found no problems associated with moonlight. Sleeping masks are effective for elevating melatonin production, which is good news for those who must sleep days or are bothered by nighttime lights. If you don't have a mask, put a pillow, a blanket or anything comfortable over your eyes when you sleep.

---

[69]   *What's Keeping You Awake at Night?*, http://brainstudy.wordpress.com/category/health/ (January 2014).

[70]   *Using iPad for Two Hours Before Bedtime Harms Your Sleep, New Study Reveals*, www.dailymail.co.uk/news/article-2272615/Using-iPad-hours-bedtime-harms-SLEEP-new-study-reveals.html (January 2014).

[71]   *In Eyes, a Clock Calibrated by Wavelengths of Light*, www.nytimes.com/2011/07/05/health/05light.html?pagewanted=all&r=0 (January 2014).

[72]   *Missing the Dark: Health Effects of Light Pollution*, www.ncbi.nlm.nih.gov/pmc/articles/PMC2627884/ (January 2014).

Although some people take melatonin supplements to aid in sleep, I do not recommend supplements except in temporary, extreme circumstances. It is much better to correct the other life imbalances that are interfering with natural melatonin production. Above all, never take sleeping pills.

THE SHOCKING TRUTH
ABOUT SLEEPING PILLS

The feeling of sleepiness when you are not in bed, and can't get there, is the meanest feeling in the world.

– Edgar Watson Howe

You may have heard the promise of happy dreams by taking a magic pill. Don't believe it. An extensive study of over 10,000 people determined that sleeping pills increase cancer risks by 35 percent. The same study showed that people taking sleeping pills were four times more likely to die (for any reason during the study) than those not taking pills who had similar health histories. Dr. Daniel Kripke, director of this Scripps Clinic study, noted, "The risk of developing lymphoma, lung, colon or prostate cancer associated with sleeping pills was greater than the effect from smoking."[73]

These facts leave me speechless. Sleeping pill users have a higher risk of getting cancer than cigarette smokers!

All sleeping pills can be addictive, despite the "non-habit forming" claims of some products. Many sleeping pill users report negative side effects including uncontrollable shaking, loss of balance, dizziness, heartburn, constipation, sleep walking and sleep driving. Hundreds of car accidents have been caused by people whose driving was impaired by sleeping pills. The residual effects of sleeping pills take up to 18 hours to dissipate. Some users don't fully wake up until it's time to go back to bed!

Sleeping pills take people through the stages of sleep at an unnatural rate, or they skip stages altogether. They do not allow people to spend the natural amount of time in Stages 4 and 5, robbing them of mind and body healing and restoration. Your body will suffer serious consequences without that healing sleep.

---

73   Alice Park, *Study: Sleeping Pills Linked with Early Death,* http://healthland.time.com/2012/02/28/study-sleeping-pills-linked-with-early-death/ (January 2014).

What sleeping pill manufacturers don't tell you is that nature's way is always safer, cheaper and more effective at restoring beautiful sleep and the natural rhythms of life. Get the other Essentials right and see how amazing your sleep will become. Sleep is unique in that it is the one essential that will likely correct itself if you get the other Essentials right. But if you don't address your sleep needs, this powerful Essential can take down all the other seven ... and fast.

SNORING AND SLEEP APNEA

> On the farm, a good day's work will give you a great night's sleep.
>
> – Frank King, Sr. (my dad!)

Snoring happens when the muscles in the roof of the mouth and throat relax, blocking the airway and vibrating audibly. Snoring is exacerbated by obesity, allergies, sickness and alcohol consumption.

When the snorer stops breathing and becomes silent for a few seconds, this is known as sleep apnea. The sleeper frequently senses that he or she is suffocating and wakes up with a loud snort or gasping sound. This may happen five times or more every hour of sleep. People with sleep apnea obviously have trouble receiving the healing benefits of Stage 4 and 5 sleep. Sleep apnea sufferers experience all the risks associated with sleep deprivation that were listed earlier.

Studies show that most sleep partners of snorers are subject to the same health risks as the snorers themselves. Researchers noted that sleep disorders caused snorers to awaken 27 times per hour while partners were awakened 21 times per hour.[74] If you are a victim of second-hand snoring, earplugs may be your best, natural remedy. If you don't like using earplugs, change your perspective, if necessary, through Tap Into Potential ("I will sleep GREAT with earplugs!").

You can eliminate or minimize the effects of sleep apnea and snoring by following the Eight Essentials. Sleep better by getting rid of excess weight and eliminating artificial foods, cosmetics and home products with toxic ingredients. Detoxify yourself with homeopathic formulas that activate

---

74   Tara Parker-Pope, *Dangers of Second-Hand Snoring: When Bedtime Is a Health Hazard*, http://online.wsj.com/article/0,,SB10691056211882000,00.html (January 2014).

the body's natural ability to cleanse itself. Exercise more, eat healthy, get your weight where it needs to be, avoid excess alcohol, don't take sleeping pills, don't smoke and avoid excess caffeine. One simple remedy is to sleep on your side rather than on your back. Prop yourself with extra pillows, if necessary. While lying in bed, practice deep, whole-body breathing as explained in the Fitness Essential. If you are experiencing serious problems with sleep apnea and snoring, see a doctor or sleep specialist.

DREAMS

Dreams are stories told by the wildly creative subconscious mind. Your sub-consciousness keeps track of everything that your senses perceive.

Imagine going to a state fair and walking as fast as you can from one end to the other, taking it all in with your senses. Your mind has just captured a "Where's Waldo" video that includes the specific face and outfit of every person within your field of vision, a detailed description of every ride and every booth, a compilation of all the smells from cotton candy to animal stalls, a soundtrack of every barker and calliope, the feel of the terrain under your feet, every cloud and bird in the sky, and much, much more. If Waldo's hat was barely visible in a crowd of a thousand people in the midway, that glimpse is stored somewhere in your memory, even though you will likely never be able to bring it to consciousness.

Your subconscious mind has access to every fact in that immense library of stored information. Your dreams can intertwine those facts with creative fiction in bizarre ways. I remember having a series of troubling dreams about venomous snakes. I was like Indiana Jones in "Raiders of the Lost Ark," surrounded by an insurmountable number of snakes. I was trapped and nearly paralyzed by them. Somebody suggested that I pick up a dream dictionary, which I did. There I read that venomous snakes represent bad people speaking poisonous accusations, which happened to be true. Someone was telling blatant lies about me at that time.

Dreams are, in part, the brain's stage for playing out some very intriguing comedies, tragedies and parodies of the immense volume of truth stored in your brain. Obviously, use common sense when making judgments based on dreams, so as not to make horribly wrong decisions based on misinterpretations. Common sense comes first. MRT may help you test for dream meanings. A dream dictionary may be helpful for identifying the

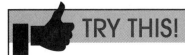
symbolic themes in your dreams, but take everything you read with a grain of salt. Dreams are quickly forgotten, so keep a notebook by your bed and jot down significant dreams during the night or in the morning.

People often have reoccurring dream themes that reveal a deep need in their lives. They might repeatedly find themselves abandoned, forgotten, embarrassed, ashamed, terrified, trapped or hunted. Sometimes the story repeats itself; other times the story is different but the emotion is the same. These may be signals of unresolved emotional needs.

In the Healing Revolution, you are destined for happy dreams. Tell people you trust about your dreams. Identify negative emotions in dreams. Use tapping to change those into the opposite, positive affirmations (e.g., "I will not be terrified in my dreams. I am safe and happy in my dreams. My dreams are guiding me into the optimal purposes of my life.").

LUCID DREAMS

Lucid dreams take the REM adventure to a higher level. Lucid dreaming simply happens when you become aware that you are dreaming. For example, you might say to yourself during a scary dream, "Wait a minute. Nothing bad can really happen to me. I'm only dreaming." Or, "Of course I can fly because this is a dream." Lucid dreaming is especially helpful in correcting negative dream emotions like fear or helplessness as you consciously recognize that it's just a dream. Sometimes you can control lucid dreams and sometimes you can't. Either way, it's extremely rewarding to be an aware observer.

Nighttime is actually good for problem-solving. The brain's creativity is enhanced and its problem-solving skills are heightened for a short period of time after awakening from dream time. Somehow the incredibly creative, seemingly random associations that happen in dreams "spill over" into real life, guiding the conscious mind in making reality decisions. Maybe you, like me, have gone to sleep with a vexing problem, then awakened with a bullet-proof solution that seems so simple. That's how your unconscious mind works while you sleep.

Make your dream time a healing time, both emotionally and physically. Your dreams belong to you. If it seems like somebody else is running the dream department, it's time you take that job back. Once you see how fun and rewarding it can be, you'll never give it up.

YOUR SLEEP SANCTUARY

We are such stuff as dreams are made on, and our little life is rounded with a sleep.

– William Shakespeare, "The Tempest"

Your bedroom is your sleep sanctuary. You will spend a third of your life in bed, so don't be too cheap when it comes to bed health and comfort. As a chiropractor, I have helped many people recover from sagging, lumpy, hard or smelly mattresses and pillows.

Lie on your side in bed with your head on your pillow and have somebody look at your back: your spine and neck should be in a straight line, from your head to the base of your spine.

Adjust the height of the pillow to achieve that straightness. If you sag in the middle, your mattress might not be firm enough.

My wife and I bought an eco-made memory foam mattress. When that didn't give us the sleep comfort we desired, we up-scaled to an adjustable air bed that allowed us to set different air pressure-controlled firmness on each side of the mattress. Avoid petrochemical-based, smelly mattresses, foam, pillows, blankets, comforters and sheets. Many people have gotten sick from breathing fumes from the chemicals and flame retardants in modern mattresses.[75] Buy a healthy, "green" mattress, or a natural rubber

---

75   *Bed and Mattress Illness Report Page*, www.chem-tox.com/guest/guestbook.html (January 2014).

mattress made from rubber trees, or cover your mattress with a food-grade polyethylene wrap.[76] Wash bed sheets in unscented, natural detergent. Buy organic cotton and wool blankets, pillows, sheets and mattress covers. Natural wool bedding may sound hot and itchy, but it is not.

A neat, orderly, dust-free bedroom, naturally lit and free of electronic devices, promotes healthy, revitalizing sleep. Feng Shui proponents suggest that the orientation of your bed contributes to restful sleep. For example, a west-facing bed may enhance feelings of contentment while an east-facing bed promotes ambition and career expansion. Some positions, such as north, north-east and south, may promote negative attitudes and emotions. Perhaps this concept relates to the magnetic orientation of the earth, since we, too, are magnetic beings. I'm intrigued by ideas like these, even if they sound strange and new. I've never been one to reject something just because science hasn't conducted laboratory tests on it yet, especially if people are seeing positive results by actually doing it. Listen to your instincts and use Muscle Reflex Testing (MRT) while facing in different directions. Experiment and try moving your bed around for a while. Maybe you'll notice some benefits to your sleep. If not, the changing perspectives will at least make life more interesting.

THE SUPER POWER OF SLEEP

Now that you have your sleep sanctuary established, it's time to unleash the super power of sleep. What is that super power? Well, it all begins with understanding your potential and purpose in life.

Know this: Your potential and purpose on this planet is much, much greater than you might think. Imagine what might happen if you actually reach your full potential!

What is that potential? You are designed to enjoy a long life of health and wholeness, and to share your unique, precious gifts with others. Keep in mind that once you are symptom-free of any negative health issues, you have not reached your stride. You have merely reached a neutral position, so to speak. You have freed yourself from the health problems that were drowning you, and you've finally pushed your nose above the surface. You are floating comfortably at sea level.

---

76   *No-Chem Bed Solutions*, www.offgassing-mattress-wraps.com/mattress-wraps.htm (January 2014).

Reach for the Sky

Bedtime is uniquely suited not only for bringing health and healing, but also for clarifying your life purpose and vision. As you fall asleep, these are some things you might seek for yourself. Reach for the sky!

▷ *Great health for your body and mind.*

▷ *Insights to create a more fulfilling life for you and your loved ones.*

▷ *Strength and freedom to leave life-destroying influences and habits behind.*

▷ *Greater clarity of your life purpose.*

▷ *"Divine appointments" (strategic relational connections) that will help you fulfill your purpose.*

▷ *Everything you need to reach your highest potential in life. Aim high, and your target might still be too low!*

This is where the fun begins. Now it's time to launch into the skies and soar with the eagles. Even if you still struggle with health issues, you can rise above the sea. Aim high, and prepare for a life of passion and purpose that far exceeds your wildest expectation. This is what I have personally experienced over and over again. Break out of the box. Smash the chains that bind you. Prepare yourself for a higher life purpose that can erase any memories of boredom or suffering that plague you from the past.

What does this have to do with sleep?

Sleep is the most powerful time of my 24-hour day, and it can be yours as well. A lot gets done in my sleep – things I can observe and things I cannot observe. I experience physical, spiritual, mental and emotional healing, problem-solving, and much more. I receive new vision and inspiration for the future. The super power of sleep enables me to struggle less and go with the flow of life more. My emotions become more balanced. I experience more positive "divine appointments" by connecting my mind and spirit to the super power of sleep.

In my unconscious state, sleep is totally working in my favor.

For example, I might go to bed wondering how to smooth over a little tension in a relationship, or how to help a patient with a so-called "incurable" disease. As I approach sleep, I make a deliberate decision not to be concerned or worried about these things. Instead, I ask for answers and solutions, often while using Tap Into Potential (TIP). I personally direct my requests toward God whom I believe is stronger and smarter than I am to fulfill my requests, although I encourage others to wholeheartedly seek their highest potential regardless of their beliefs.

The next morning – or more likely, in a random moment several days later – I receive a supernatural new outlook on the problem or challenge which faced me. Or I am led to a chance meeting or divine appointment that positively changes my world. You, too, can go far beyond your own abilities by turning to a Higher Power.

Expect terrific results in this process. Whatever your target is, you are probably not aiming high enough. Reach for the sky as you consider your highest purpose in life. Build upon your passions, and the unique gifts you have that will bless other people and make the world a better place.

Pursue the new-you with all your heart and soul.

If you are inactive, adding a 10 minute walk every day could improve your likelihood of a good night's sleep.

– Dr. Max Hirshkowitz, "Exercise Key to Good Sleep," ScienceDaily.com, March 4, 2013.

Desire an amazing, powerful new potential and purpose for your life.
Believe that you can and will experience this transforming power.
Become *the new you … as you happily slip off to sleep.*

Give it a try. This just might be the key to unlock the changes you have desired to see in your life. These changes might not happen overnight, but see if this attitude of super sleep doesn't totally transform your life. Your path to a higher purpose and potential can, indeed, become a dream come true. Your bed becomes like a raft in a river of awesome possibilities, and there's no saying in which amazing new land you will awaken in the morning.

DR. KING'S HAPPY BEDTIME ADVICE

These are some simple recommendations to improve your bedtime hours:
- *Avoid overeating anytime, but especially in the evening. It is best to have your last meal at least three hours before bedtime.*
- *Naturally avoid stimulants like caffeine and nicotine.*
- *Helpful tools for neutralizing distractions include ear plugs, sleeping*

masks and a fan or other device to generate white noise if absolutely necessary.

◆ Open the window, if the weather allows, since indoor air is generally not as healthy as fresh, outdoor air. The gases given off by many building materials and household chemicals are bad for health.

◆ Make any necessary changes that will enhance your sleep sanctuary, as explained earlier.

◆ Turn the lights down low and avoid fluorescent and blue light. Avoid watching TV or an electronic screen before bedtime.

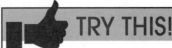

TRY THIS!

TIP: Tap Yourself to Sleep
TIP is explained on page 201.

• Tap yourself to sleep while improvising statements like, "I release all the concerns of today. I am free of all cares. I can sleep well now. I will breathe deep. I will sleep deep. I'm lying in God's cradle of care. God is working on my behalf, even more than all I can think or ask." Continue to improvise until you are sound asleep.

Avoid video violence that can cause bad dreams, especially for children.

◆ Turn off or remove all electro-magnetic field sources that might interfere with your sleep time. Some studies suggest that EMFs from power lines, electricity substations, home electrical wiring, Wi-Fi Internet, cell phones, computers, home appliances, microwave ovens, fluorescent lights, hair dryers and electric blankets can cause anything from sleep disturbances to chronic disease. Keep cell phones, computers and electronic devices out of your bedroom.[77]

◆ Enjoy a soothing cup of nighttime, herbal tea such as chamomile before going to bed.

◆ If you have trouble easing your mind, try using TIP to relax. Meditate on beautiful music, poetry, photos, landscapes or writings. Memorize some of your favorite inspirational writings and meditate on each word as you lie in bed.

◆ Refuse to let all the frantic concerns of the day invade your evening hours. Save heavy discussions for the next day. Release unresolved problems to your Higher Power. Let go of any negative experiences, emotions or disappointment. As you bunk down for the night, make a conscious decision to trade in the day's junk for generous portions of love, joy,

---

77   More will be said about EMFs in Essential #6: Nature.

peace, compassion, tolerance, forgiveness and beauty.

◆ Take a hot shower, bath or sauna. The relaxing rise in body temperature tells your body systems to prepare to sleep. Visualize all the problems, worries and negative emotions of the day being washed down the drain. Meditate on positive attitudes as you head for bed.

◆ A sea salt or Epsom salt bath is one of my favorite calming therapies, with natural magnesium and 80 other essential minerals. After bathing, take a little time to allow the minerals to naturally dry on your body and be absorbed through your skin.

◆ If you wake in the middle of the night with a worry or concern that you just can't shake, write it down and include any nocturnal insights, however crazy they might seem. Then rest assured that you've done all you can. Release your concerns to a Higher Power, knowing that your problem will be in good hands. Channel your thoughts to things of peace and beauty. Sometimes situations seem much worse at night than they really are.

◆ Yoga is an effective relaxation technique that aides in sleep. Slowly tense and relax each muscle group in your body, starting with your toes and gradually travelling through your feet, ankles, calves, knees, thighs, buttocks, belly and so forth. Practice full-body breathing while doing this routine. You will probably find yoga to be so relaxing that you will never get to your scalp before falling sound asleep.

◆ As mentioned earlier, regular exercise is one of the best ways to earn a good night's sleep, but don't exercise too close to bedtime or you might find it difficult to fall asleep.

◆ In case you were wondering, sex is good for sleep, particularly after an orgasm when the body releases happy endorphins that promote sleep by making you feel calm and satisfied.

◆ Never take sleeping pills because of the many destructive side-effects that were previously mentioned. Consider taking natural sleep remedies like valerian, kava kava, hops, homeopathic remedies or chamomile. Try tapping to change negative sleep patterns.

All Eight Essentials are intricately connected. Our free, Whole Person Appraisal at www.DrFrankKing.com will help you identify additional, practical, life-affirming choices to make in all Eight Essentials of life. Make good choices all day long and you will reap the rewards of a good night's sleep. Natural is better – it's a principle to live by.

If you are not experiencing the sleep you need, take back your sleep!

Desire the perfect, natural sleep.
Believe that you can become a super-natural sleeper.
Become a super-natural sleeper.

Now enjoy the restorative powers and amazing dreams of super-natural sleep.

SELF-EVALUATION
SLEEP

My Life-Destroying Choices (e.g.: using sleeping pills, negative exercise and media habits that impact sleep)	**My Life-Affirming Choices** (e.g.: make sleep a priority, eliminate things that keep me awake at night)
1	1
2	2
3	3
4	4
5	5
6	6
7	7

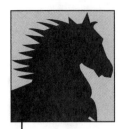

Lady's Story:
The Arabian Mare

Lady was a gorgeous Arabian mare, but she was what we called a "hard keeper." She couldn't stay out in the pasture with the other mares because she was nervous, anti-social and she'd lose too much weight. So we kept her in the stall at night and give her more personal, hands-on attention.

One morning I went out to check on Lady and she was gone! Her stall door was open and I could see that she'd gotten into the feed.

It looks like she ate everything she possibly could, I thought, looking at the nearly-empty feed bin. *She must have really packed it in. But where did she go?*

I followed her trail to the door that opened to the pasture.

She went out to pasture.

I left the stable in search of Lady. It didn't take me long to find her out in the pasture ... and she was a wreck.

Lady lay helpless on the ground. It was clear that she had been down for hours. She had been unable to get off her side, so she had tossed her head up and down in the dirt and rubbed the hair off large parts of her head, neck and body. She could barely claw the earth with her front hooves.

I knew quite a bit about animal health, having cared for animals on the farm and worked with a large-animal veterinarian in high school and college. Still, I called a trusted veterinarian friend who confirmed my fears.

"She's got colic," he said. "All that grain she ate is rotting her gut. It's a hopeless case, Frank. We'll have to put her down."

I had no problem with the diagnosis but I challenged his recommendation.

"I'm not gonna put her down."

"This horse need not suffer," he insisted. "She can barely move, Frank, and she'll never recover. Everybody knows that colic kills horses when it gets this intense. You can put her out of her misery right here and now."

"I can't do it," I said, "at least not until I've tried everything I possibly can. She's still got a fighting chance, and I'm going to help her take it."

In truth, I couldn't see any fight left in her. She looked as bad a case as I've ever seen.

"All right, Frank," said the vet. "You're a stubborn one. Just let me leave this with you." He handed me a syringe with the measured dose of euthanizing drug. "You'll be needing it soon enough."

I put the killing medicine in the refrigerator, then called out the supporting troops. Four of us grown men got down beside Lady.

Her coat was wringing wet with sweat from the colic. The bald side of her looked pitiful where she had rubbed it against the ground. Getting her up on her feet was her only hope of survival. If she remained on the ground, gas and fluid would settle in her gut, she would get pneumonia and she'd eventually die.

We rocked Lady, stroked her, pushed her and pulled her until we were finally able to get her up to her feet. The other guys held her while I got her to drink a little water. Then I administered some homeopathic colic medicine. I gave her four doses the first hour, and then one dose per hour after that.

I'm not sure how, but she was still standing when night fell. I visited her repeatedly through the night and kept giving her the natural remedy. Her fever began to break. By the end of the next day, she was walking and feeling much better. Within a few days she was back to normal, except for the hair that took some weeks to grow back.

In reality, Lady turned out better than ever before. She became an easy keeper and we kept her out in the field all summer long. She lost her nervousness, becoming perfectly calm and pleasantly socialized with the other horses. What's more, we bred her with the king of English horses – a rare hackney stallion, the kind that knights used for jousting and queens used for carriages. Lady birthed several breathtakingly beautiful foals which fetched a high price in the horse lover's market.

I always loved that phenomenal horse and was extremely grateful that we never had to put her down. She reminds me that the Healing Revolution can impact our animal companions, just as surely as it helps you and me.

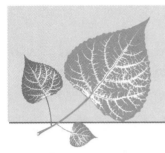

ESSENTIAL #6:
NATURE

I frequently tramped eight or ten miles through the deepest snow to keep an appointment with a beech-tree, or a yellow birch, or an old acquaintance among the pines.

– Henry David Thoreau,
"Winter Visitors"

Nature is such a beautifully healing and energizing force. I remember stepping out onto our wooden deck on a balmy Saturday morning in April. I took one deep breath and nature did its wonder-working magic on me. The energizing warmth of the morning sun transformed me. I literally felt lighter as the stresses of the week seemed to drop like scales from my body. So much can happen in nature, even when it seems like nothing is happening.

I took another breath. I stretched my back like a cat and felt the breeze on my face.

Baa … Baa …

Sheep nibbled their way through the neighbor's pasture. Yellow daffodils were beginning to pop up along the fence line. My gaze followed the fence to the forest, skipping across a distant pasture on ancient boulders, to the ridgelines of seven Appalachian Mountain ranges, each fading into a paler shade of blue. I began to sense that something incredible was happening … something that men and women have intuitively known and experienced since the beginning of time.

A cleansing, healing, bioenergetic force was renewing me from the outside-in. I was experiencing what homeopathy's founder Samuel Hahnemann called the life force, or what Taoists and acupuncturists call chi. One of my favorite ways to rest and recharge my depleted physical and mental accounts is simply to commune with nature, alone or with others.

On that particular Appalachian springtime morning, I spent some time alone in the woods, my feet and my thoughts wandering with no particular destination in mind. Mainly I was "busy" overseeing the greening of pastures and blooming of flowers.

"Hey Dad," called my 12-year-old daughter from the house. "Do you wanna play Hunger Games with me?"

"Yeah!" I shouted. "Sounds fun."

Hunger Games is our pretend survival game where we hide sacks of provisions in the woods for each other to find, which include things like fish crackers, towel bandages and natural medical supplies. My daughter usually wins because she's such a fast runner and a good hider. This time, however, I surprised her with a slick move that she didn't think her old man of 60-years-old still had in him. We were negotiating a truce to the war across a fence, while I casually rested my hands on the top rail. Suddenly I kicked a leg up, used my arm as a lever and vaulted over the fence just like I used to do when I was a kid on the farm. I caught her totally off guard and put her in a headlock. We both struggled and fell to the ground with big smiles on our faces. The Hunger Games ended with us laughing like school kids and eating the last of our provisions.

SPRINGTIME IS AN ATTITUDE

Ever since I was a boy, I have loved springtime. It's such an amazing time of life and growth. I see each new blade of grass and each budding bush and tree as miracles of life. And they are! The springtime forces are so strong. The new grasses aren't like those in the autumn that shrink back and surrender to the threat of winter. The springtime grasses are hardly budged by the frost.

That's what happens when we get in touch with nature, when the energy of springtime courses through our veins. The sunshine, the breeze, the rain and the energy revive and invigorate us. We invite these forces to strengthen us, making us more resistant to disease and depression. This positive healing energy is even stronger than our chromosomes, as the science of epigenetics teaches us. This life force is powerful enough to shut down negative genetic expressions, while enhancing the positive, life-giving tendencies.

Springtime is an attitude. Have you ever seen that old woman with the mischievous twinkle in her eye? ... or the codger who always has a wisecrack or a sly trick up his sleeve? It's like Dr. Paul Bragg, the 80-year-old guy who inspired me while standing on his head. These kinds of people choose not to define themselves by the aches and limitations of the so-called "autumn" of life. They have discovered how to make springtime a personal attitude of life.

The life force of nature renews and revitalizes us perpetually – through the years – like when my son and I enjoy apples or figs from the trees I planted twenty-some years ago ... or when we watch our yaks or bison birth a new generation of young into our pastures. That force seems to gain force and intensity through the years, like a rolling snowball. It becomes more fulfilling than I can describe. We are truly designed to enjoy the results of our labor in nature as they grow, develop, and bear young, fruit or seed. This is true whether you are raising buffalo on the range, or if you simply grow one small tomato plant on the balcony of your third-floor apartment.

That's something the long-living Blue Zone people know instinctively. They never lost the enduring intensity of nature, as they tend grapevines and mend fences that were established by their ancestors. They rise each morning with brother sun and end the day with sister moon. They walk on grassy hillsides overlooking the great, blue sea, same as their fathers and mothers before them.

This is an attitude that we must recover in the Healing Revolution. It's not easy to push back the city, the highway, the job, the TV and all the crud that tries to dilute and pollute our little green square of paradise. Take it back! However you can – in even the smallest way – nurture and protect nature in your life. Plant a seed – in your heart AND in the ground. Give those seedlings room to grow. Make this an attitude of gratitude for the rest of your life. Plan to nurture and enjoy this plant for many, many years to come.

The attitude of nature brings a perpetual revitalization, an ongoing renewal, an enduring regeneration. This is the renewing potential of nature.

WHAT IS NATURE?

Nature is the natural world. Its vast panoramas span oceans, deserts and mountain ranges. Its intimate beauty is found in autumn leaves, mushrooms and delicate snowflakes. Nature is a rugged trek into the Alaskan wilderness. It is a momentary pause to watch a swaying branch or a busy squirrel beside a city sidewalk.

Human beings have historically, in diverse ways, woven nature into their life rhythms, tied closely as they were to the land. Regrettably, modernity's machine has ripped through this fabric and cut the ties. Sadly, we are still reeling from the collision. Our ancestors didn't need to be told to stop and smell the roses. Unfortunately, we need constant reminders. Nature is one more life Essential to take back if we are to experience healthy and fulfilled lives.

Some powerful ways to connect with nature include:

- *walking barefoot on the grass,*
- *lying on your back while watching the clouds in the sky,*
- *pressing a seed into the moist earth,*
- *sleeping in a forest, or*
- *washing your face in a stream.*

The best remedy for those who are afraid, lonely or unhappy is to go outside, somewhere where they can be quite alone with the heavens, nature and God. Because only then does one feel that all is as it should be and that God wishes to see people happy, amidst the simple beauty of nature. As long as this exists ... there will always be comfort for every sorrow, whatever the circumstances may be.

– Anne Frank, "The Diary of a Young Girl"

You need not take a two-hour drive to the country to experience nature. Doctor Sunshine is waiting right outside your door with a natural prescription for your health. Breathe deep of vitamin O – oxygen – as you commune with nature. If all you have is ten minutes today for a walk in the garden, take it. Restoration, renewal, revival and rehabilitation happen when we unplug ourselves from modernity's machine and weave ourselves back into the nurturing fabric of nature's web.

NATURE NURTURES US; WE NURTURE NATURE

A polar bear transported from his natural environment above the Arctic Circle to the Death Valley of California won't survive long there in the Mojave Desert. A fish dies without water. We can't survive without our connection to the sunlight, the air, the soil and the earth.

In the nutrition chapter, I warned against gathering berries and plants that grow along highways because of the contaminating pollutants. Research also shows that when people live close to busy traffic, their risk of atherosclerosis (clogged arteries) increases. Air pollution is not the only problem; the noise of traffic also negatively affects health.[78]

The more disconnected we become with the earth, the more we inhibit our body's natural ability to heal. Natural is better … it's a principle to live by. We were designed to live in synch with our environment. Synchronicity means aligning values, function and purpose with the days, weeks, months, seasons, tides, energies, migrations and natural rhythms of life.

The holistic health movement is linked hand-in-glove with a green earth. Sustainable living extends seamlessly from healthy hearts, minds and souls to the streets of our cities and the paths of our forests. The Eight Essentials that are good for you and me are also good for the earth. On the other hand, cultural, social, agricultural, scientific, political and personal decisions that are made solely for economic or pragmatic reasons usually end up being catastrophic to both health and the environment. This should come as no surprise. The life-giving principles of nature are not lopsided in their benefits. Our lifestyle choices could not be good and right if they benefited people while raping the earth.

An awesome benefit of a natural, healthy lifestyle is that it restores peace and connectedness between us and our environment. The living earth beneath our feet is a patient teacher if we will only listen and learn. Nature nurtures us, and we nurture nature when our priorities are in order.

---

78   American Thoracic Society, *Air Pollution and Noise Pollution Increase Cardiovascular Risk*, www.sciencedaily.com/releases/2013/05/130520142745.htm (January 2014).

Nature also nurtures our positive gene expressions. Epigenetics – the study of changes in gene expression – proves that you are not destined to inherit the negative genetic tendencies that run in your family. Your siblings might all die of cancer, but you are NOT destined to go down the same way. Nature is an important Essential for reprogramming those gene expressions. The more you connect with nature – and the more healthy lifestyle choices you make – the greater results you will experience. Nature nurtures you by enhancing your positive gene expressions.

INDOOR ZOMBIES

Zombies despise the sunshine. They abhor the fresh air. They don't enjoy the beautiful flowers and trees. Unfortunately, many people today are becoming like indoor zombies.

The Environmental Protection Agency (EPA) says that Americans spend about 90% of their time indoors, where pollutants are two to five times higher than outside. Spending time outside raises Vitamin D levels, strengthens bones, alleviates stress and lowers susceptibility to heart disease, diabetes and other health problems.[79]

I am especially concerned about children. There was a time when people took it for granted that kids would spend large amounts of time outdoors. According to a recent Kaiser Family Foundation study, "8 to 18 year-olds devote an average of 7 hours and 38 minutes (7:38) to using entertainment media across a typical day (more than 53 hours a week)."[80] In contrast,

> *A village is not complete, unless it have these trees to mark the season in it. They are important, like the town-clock. A village that has them not will not be found to work well. It has a screw loose, an essential part is wanting … A village needs these innocent stimulants of bright and cheering prospects to keep off melancholy and superstition.*
>
> *– Henry David Thoreau, "Autumnal Tints"*

---

79   *Health Benefits*, www.nwf.org/Be-Out-There/Why-Be-Out-There/Health-Benefits.aspx (January 2014).
80   Victoria J. Rideout, Ulla G. Foehr, and Donald F. Roberts, *Generation M2: Media in the Lives of 8- to 18-Year-Olds*, (Menlo Park, CA: Kaiser Family Foundation, 2010); http://kff.org/other/report/generation-m2-media-in-the-lives-of-8-to-18-year-olds/ (January 2014).

children spend only 4 to 7 minutes outside in unstructured playtime each day. Research shows that outdoor play increases fitness, improves vision, reduces ADHD symptoms and improves test and critical thinking scores.

Too many people today have forgotten the refreshing feel of tender grass under bare feet. It's no wonder that obesity, type 2 diabetes and other inflammatory conditions have become like a black plague to sedentary people of the 21st century. Let us reap the benefits of connecting ourselves and our children to the earth.

GROUND YOURSELF

Our scientific understanding of bioenergetic forces and how they interact with the earth is new and not well developed, but it is growing. We do know that the earth is like a giant battery, alive with natural energies that charge, energize, nurture and heal.

Humans are electrical beings as well. Every muscle is stimulated by electricity. Trillions of cells continuously interact with each other and they also interact with the electrical grid of the earth. Problems occur when brain-to-muscle impulses get blocked or mixed. Similarly, problems occur when body-to-earth connections are disrupted.

Our ancestors worked, played and lived in closer connection to the earth's energy than we do. We wear rubber-soled shoes that prevent us from grounding with the earth, causing an unhealthy build-up of static electromagnetic fields (EMFs) within our bodies. We sleep on beds that act as insulators from the natural energies in the ground. We have ungrounded ourselves in high rise apartments and office cubicles lighted by fluorescent lights. We have unplugged ourselves from the electric earth.

Are you relaxing in a chair right now? Are you wearing comfortable shoes or sandals? Are you reclining in bed? Wherever you are, if you connect yourself to a volt-ohm meter – a device that measures electrical charges – you will most certainly see that your body has a small positive charge. Your positive charge will be even higher if you are surrounded by

> *Children spend only 4 to 7 minutes outside in unstructured playtime each day, while sitting over 7 ½ hours in front of electronic devices.*

electronic devices and electric lighting. Now, if you touch a grounded metal appliance or cable – or if you take your shoes off and stand barefoot on the ground – your electrical charge will drop to zero, or close to it.

The problem, according to the authors of the book *Earthing*, is that most of us spend the vast majority of time ungrounded, holding this unnatural positive charge in our body. We are disconnected from the earth, leaving us "vulnerable and prone to dysfunction, inflammation-related disease and accelerated aging."[81] They advocate "earthing," which means grounding to the earth by walking barefoot, wearing non-insulating footwear and by sleeping on the ground or with a natural bed-to-earth grounding connection.

The earth is more than just a patch of dirt. It is a source of healing; a battery to recharge bioenergy. The Blue Zone people who live meaningful lives into their second century spend lots of time outdoors. They plant gardens and care for animals in the open air. Walking is their common form of transportation. They commune with Doctor Sunshine and Mother Nature. They breathe deep of vitamin O. Their closeness to the earth unquestionably contributes to their longevity. Reconnecting with nature is a wonderful, life-giving Essential of the Healing Revolution.

GOING BAREFOOT

Take a moment to look at your shoe collection. If you are anything like I was when I first began to explore earthing, I was surprised to see that all of my shoes were rubber, plastic or synthetic-soled. These types of shoes are insulators, disconnecting us from the electrical energies of the earth.

> In every walk with nature one receives far more than he seeks.
>
> – *John Muir*

Besides the insulating properties, many shoes today constrict feet in unhealthy ways. When I was six years old, my brother boosted me up on a pony in our pasture. I clung on for dear life, riding bareback with nothing to hold onto but the mane. When the pony ran under a large thorn tree and brushed me off like a fly, I crashed to the ground, using my left arm to brace my fall. That's when a stabbing pain told me something wasn't right. I gasped to find a brand-new bend in my

---

81   Stephen Sinatra, Clinton Ober and Martin Zucker, *Earthing* (Laguna Beach, CA: Basic Health Publications, Inc., 2010).

forearm that hinged like my wrist, but with a clunking sound. It was a compound fracture. The doctor immobilized my arm in a plaster cast that was bent 90-degrees at the elbow for six weeks. When the cast finally came off, I was unable to straighten my arm. It took me nearly a week of stretching before I could finally straighten it again.

Shoes act like plaster casts over the 26 bones of the foot. The muscles, tendons and joints are restricted and weakened when they are over-supported and immobilized by restrictive shoes. I am not an advocate for no shoes, all the time, but I am against all shoes, all the time. We obviously need foot protection from the hazards of modern life, glass, burrs, thistles, ice and snow. Additionally, athletic shoes provide necessary support and protection for more extreme conditions, or for the impact of walking or running on hard surfaces.

Comfortable, affordable, leather-soled shoes for men, women and children are difficult to find. Dance shoes and men's dress shoes are available in leather, but they generally are not practical for everyday use. Leather moccasins are a better alternative if you can find them.

Recent innovations in footwear styles are offering some promise for better health and a barefoot feel. Some of these styles are roomier and more flexible than conventional shoes. Others fit like a glove. I suggest trying different styles to find what works best for you. Be aware that feet typically swell during the day, so try on shoes later in the day to find the best, most natural fit.

Going barefoot, at least part of the time, is a wonderful way to be grounded. It allows harmful electromagnetic charges to be transmitted from your body into the ground. Go barefoot as much as you can around the house. As you begin integrating barefoot time into your daily schedule, you may experience some soreness, especially in the arches. This is a

> *Verily these maples are cheap preachers, permanently settled, which preach their half-century and century, ay and century-and-a-half sermons, with constantly increasing unction and influence, ministering to many generations of men; and the least we can do is to supply them with suitable colleagues as they grow infirm.*
>
> *– Henry David Thoreau, "Autumnal Tints"*

normal part of the strengthening process. Begin slowly, especially if you are overweight or have a history of foot problems. Naturally, consult with your doctor if you have troubling foot problems.

Take your barefoot journey outdoors. Begin on green grass, but steer clear of chemically treated lawns to avoid absorbing harmful toxins through your skin.[82] The beach is one of the best places to bare your feet, on the hard sand where the waves come in. The negative ions from the water and the salt from the sea are extra benefits of walking along the ocean. Walk outside for just ten minutes a day and see if you don't begin to feel better. The morning dew and frost are morning super-chargers!

NEGATIVE IONS, POSITIVE PEOPLE

Close your eyes and imagine the powerful roar of a waterfall. Feel the mist on your face. Imagine the crashing surf of the ocean and the foam at your feet. Imagine the feel of a passing thunderstorm. These experiences leave you energized, don't they? You feel supercharged and relaxed, with a heightened sense of awareness.

This feeling is common in nature. Even a momentary pause under a leafy tree or the song of a bird and the breath of wind can jump-start the recharging and restoration process. It happens instantly ... almost miraculously.

Negative ions are part of the electrical charge of the earth. They are naturally created in the intersection of sunlight, wind, trees, earth and water. The feeling of heightened awareness and contentment in the presence of these ions is not a myth. Negative ions increase the flow of oxygen to the brain, resulting in higher alertness, increased wakefulness and increased brainpower.[83]

Negative ions improve the mood of people who are clinically depressed. Not only do they stimulate feel-good brain chemistry, but they improve the body's reaction to allergenic substances.

On the other hand, positive ions deplete the body's energy and leave the mind more susceptible to depression. Positive ions are concentrated in air and water pollution, hydrocarbon exhausts, toxins, dust, pet dander and

---

82   Related to that, be careful where you let your pets play, since too many pets are getting sick from fertilizers, herbicides and pesticides.

83   *Negative Ions Create Positive Vibes*, www.webmd.com/balance/features/negative-ions-create-positive-vibes (January 2014).

household cleaning products. Air conditioners, cell phones, televisions, microwaves and computers emit a continuous stream of positive ions.

Because the cells of the human body carry a negative electrical charge, we tend to attract the unhealthy positive ions from the environment. "Opposites attract," as the laws of physics state. This tendency, if not kept in proper balance by increasing exposure to negative ions, spells danger for people in need of a Healing Revolution.

Blowing up the TV and moving to an off-the-grid farm is not for everyone, although that style has suited some people quite well. A more workable solution for most people is to increase exposure to negative ions while decreasing exposure to positive ones.

***To increase your exposure
to negative ions:***

◆ *Open the window and turn off the air conditioner.*
◆ *Go for a walk, in sunshine or rain.*
◆ *Take your work outside for a few minutes a day, onto the lawn or to a park.*
◆ *Use a salt lamp, which emits negative ions, instead of conventional lighting.*
◆ *Go barefoot, ground your bed and furniture, and implement other suggestions from the book* Earthing.
◆ *Set up a small indoor fountain.*
◆ *Shut off the computer and other electronic devices when not in use.*
◆ *Step outside for a short Energizing Technique (ET) break several times during your work day.*

👍 **TRY THIS!**

MRT and TIP:
Take Nature Back
*(see Essential #8 for
help using MRT and TIP)*

• *Use MRT to test statements relating to nature and health such as, "My indoor air is healthy. I need to open the windows and doors more. I love the sunshine. I love walking barefoot. Bugs don't bug me. I love being outdoors." Make lifestyle changes in any areas that test weak.*

• *Use TIP to give you strength and motivation to make the necessary lifestyle changes. Directly address your TV, computer, media and indoor habits. Address your fears and obstacles of being outdoors more.*

YOUR FUTURE LOOKS BRIGHT

Your future looks exceptionally bright, especially if you regularly spend time with Doctor Sunshine. Natural light is great for your health. Unfortunately, many people have darkened their destiny, becoming like solar-phobic zombies who abhor the light. They are not much like their ancestors, many of whom spent 10 or more hours a day outside hunting, tending crops and performing manual labor. I have no problem with Thomas Edison's "bright idea" – the incandescent light bulb – except when it keeps us excessively indoors, away from the life-giving sunlight and the natural rhythms of life and light.

> *Light is nothing short of miraculous. Light makes our world luminous, dazzles our senses and quietly controls the chemical tides in our bodies.*
>
> **– George Brainard, "The Healing Light"**

With the average child staring at an electronic device for over seven hours each day, it's no wonder that ADHD, obesity and a host of other childhood problems have risen to epidemic rates. With adults spending less than 30 minutes outside in the sunlight, it's no wonder we feel so out of rhythm and out of sync. Our bodies are dependent on the full spectrum of light wavelengths. The Healing Revolution is illuminated by generous doses of natural light.

Up to 20 percent of Americans experience seasonal affective disorder (SAD), brought on by shorter days and less sunshine in the winter months. SAD is "characterized by moodiness, depression, cravings for simple carbohydrates, weight gain, fatigue and melancholy ... The affliction tends to be more prominent in young people and women."[84] Here are a few suggestions for beating the winter blues:

◆ *Walk or exercise outside each day, getting as much sunshine as possible.*
◆ *Use full-spectrum indoor lights, to replicate natural light.*
◆ *Seek professional help through cognitive behavioral therapy, if SAD persists.*
◆ *Take steps to improve your life in all Eight Essentials. For example, poor sleep, lack of exercise and poor diet all cause SAD to worsen.*

---

84   *Beat the Winter Blues with These Tips*, www.naturalnews.com/z042817_winter_blues_seasonal_affective_disorder_mental_health.html (January 2014).

ELECTRONIC DEVICES AND EMFS

As mentioned earlier, the average child spends 7 ½ hours a day – or 53 hours a week – in front of electronic media. National Public Radio reports, "Every major gaming company worldwide … has in place a fully developed business intelligence unit … They are trying to find out, what can they tweak to make us play just a bit longer? What would make the game more fun? What can get us to spend some money inside a game and buy something? … The idea is to make gamers uncomfortable, frustrate them, take away their powers, crush their forts, and then, at the last second, offer them a way out for a price."[85] Many parents feel totally helpless, unable to get their children away from the screens. This only underscores the urgent need for parents to start early in life, showing kids the amazing, life-giving value of nature … and all Eight Essentials of life.

Meanwhile, if you are like the average adult, you will spend about 34 hours in front of a television or personal electronic device each week. Additionally, you may cuddle up to the electromagnetic field (EMF) of a cell phone that lives in your pocket or purse for much of the day. You might mop up EMFs from computers, printers, telecommunication equipment and indoor lighting for a third of the day at work. You may spend significant time in the vicinity of home and kitchen appliances. You may live or commute near high-voltage electrical lines, and perhaps even go to sleep within snuggling distance of these super-sized EMF transmitters.

Research into the long-term effects of EMFs is sparse, primarily due to their recent introduction into our daily lives, and because of the shallow assumption that "they must be harmless." Nevertheless, international studies are now confirming some disturbing negative effects of EMFs on human health. Unbiased research is muddled by a powerful coalition of cell phone and electronic device manufacturers whose expanding markets rest upon the claim that EMFs are harmless. Studies funded by the cell phone industry are two to three times more likely than independent studies to find that EMFs have "no effect" on human health. Strong voices may try to downplay the harms, but nobody is suggesting that EMFs are good for health.[86]

---

85   Steve Henn, *How Video Games Are Getting Inside Your Head And Wallet*, www.npr.org/blogs/alltechconsidered/2013/10/30/241449067/how-video-games-are-getting-inside-your-head-and-wallet (October 29, 2013).
86   *Cell Phone Dangers: Dr. Devron Davis*, http://citizensforsafetechnology.org/Cell-Phone-Dangers-Dr-Devra-Davis,8,2263 (January 2014).

The case of one young woman with breast cancer became especially noteworthy when she revealed her curious habit of carrying her cell phone in her bra. Cancer researchers discovered that the distribution of the cancerous cells lined up perfectly with the EMF transmissions from her cell phone. [87]

The International Agency for Research on Cancer determined that cell phones are "possibly" carcinogenic to humans. They recommend using "hands free" devices, or texting instead of talking on the phone, since EMF exposure is reduced substantially the further the device is from the head and brain. The World Health Organization reports that about 4.6 billion people globally use cell phones.[88]

EMFs may cause cancer by interfering with the body's DNA repair mechanism. Children are at greater risk, since their brain cells are still in the developmental stage. The French government has recognized this fact and banned cell phone advertising to children under 12. Other European countries are taking similar measures to minimize child cell phone usage, to reduce cell phone radiation levels and to make it mandatory to include hands-free earphones with all phones sold. Several insurance companies have refused to insure cell phone manufacturers against health-related claims.[89]

For the best health, limit your exposure to cell phones and electronic devices. Use a hands-free earphone and microphone, especially if you spend a lot of time talking on your cell phone. As mentioned in the Sleep Essential chapter, people exposed to LED screens and fluorescent lights before bedtime experience additional risks of sleep disruption, melatonin deficiency and many other short- and long-term health problems.

MAL-ILLUMINATION

Modern technologies have allowed people to disregard the seasons and work long and hard all year round. Only recently have we begun to unearth some unanticipated, negative consequences to this fact of life after the Industrial Revolution. Researchers suggest that the human body

---

87   Ibid.

88   *Electromagnetic Fields and Public Health: Mobile Phones*, World Health Organization Fact sheet #193, June 2011, www.who.int/mediacentre/factsheets/fs193/en/.

89   Devra Dutton, *Disconnect: The Truth About Cell Phone Radiation* (New York: Dutton, 2010).

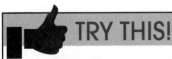

TRY THIS!

MRT: Getting Enough Light

MRT is explained on page 197

- *Get a baseline MRT.*
- *Blindfold your eyes to block out all light for 2 minutes.*
- *Repeat MRT. If your muscle weakens, it is an indication that you might need more sunlight.*

is programmed to store more fat on long days than on short ones. As the days shorten in the fall, animals and humans are supposed to eat more, storing up fat for the lean, winter months. I have observed this first hand with bison and other farm animals.

Kenneth Ceder and Robert Mathias, coauthors of *Mal-Illumination: The Silent Epidemic*, write, "Artificial lights trick the body into thinking every day, year-round, is the season to eat a lot and gain weight … Long hours of light cause insulin release to store extra carbohydrates as fat and cholesterol to have something to live on when summer is over."[90] Unfortunately, summer never ends, or so the body believes.

The authors further explain, "Light is to mal-illumination as food is to malnutrition."[91] Light governs our biorhythms. Natural sunlight is life-affirming and artificial light is not.

Your best prescription is probably not to turn off all artificial lights, but to maintain a healthy balance. Make sure your time spent in artificial light is offset by a generous amount of time outdoors. Limit your screen time and especially avoid it just before going to bed. Replace your normal light bulbs with full spectrum bulbs, which more faithfully replicate the natural rays of the sun. Hopefully you have not lost a natural love for playing outside and exploring the great outdoors. Keep these things in balance and healing will revolutionize your life.

SKIN CANCER AND THE SUNSHINE VITAMIN

Suppose you are enjoying an African safari. Suddenly you see a sad sight: an elephant lying in the dirt, struggling in the final throes of death. Worse yet, he is attacked by three vultures and a skinny hyena. Moments later, the once-invincible beast lies dead.

---

90 Kenneth Ceder and Robert Mathias, *Mal-Illumination, The Silent Epidemic*, (Santa Barbara, CA: Circadian Health Institute, 2007), p. 13. www.malillumination.org/E-book.html.

91 Ibid, p. 2.

Who killed the elephant? It is true that the vultures and hyena played a part in its demise, but it is unlikely that they could conquer this kingly creature unless it had already been weakened by disease or injury.

The same is true with sunlight and skin cancer. If you are weakened and at a high risk of getting cancer, it is wise advice to avoid excess sun. Still, the average person perhaps does more harm than good by continually covering up with hats, shawls, sunglasses and sunscreen. That is like the mighty elephant cowering in a cave for fear of the vulture's little beak.

> *They took all the trees*
> *Put 'em in a tree museum*
> *And they charged the people*
> *A dollar and a half just to see 'em*
> *Don't it always seem to go*
> *That you don't know what you've*
> *got 'til it's gone*
> *They paved paradise*
> *And put up a parking lot.*
>
> **– Joni Mitchell,**
> **"Big Yellow Taxi"**

Here's a shocking fact that was brought to light by the Environmental Working Group: Most sunscreens contain carcinogenic chemicals like oxybenzone or retinyl palmitate that are absorbed through the skin into the body.[92] People topically apply a cancer-producing substance because they are afraid of getting cancer. How much sense does that make? What's more, research shows that insufficient full-spectrum light contributes to weight gain, fatigue, depression, headaches, pain, hormonal imbalances, sleep disorders, PMS, lowered immune responses, a troubling assortment of conditions linked to vitamin D deficiency, and yes, even cancer.[93]

Sunlight is so healthy that it helps *prevent* cancer, especially by increasing the body's production of vitamin D. It is too bad that our culture has added sun-phobia to its other unhealthy habits. This leads people to a vicious cycle of less exposure to the sun, less vitamin D production, using carcinogenic sunscreens and a higher risk of cancer.

Thankfully the sunshine vitamin, vitamin D, is free for everyone, it is readily available in great abundance and the manufacturing plant is only skin-deep. Direct exposure to sunlight activates production of this vitamin

92   Danielle Delorto, *Avoid Sunscreens with Potentially Harmful Ingredients, Group Warns*, www.cnn.com/2012/05/16/health/sunscreen-report (January 2014).

93   Ceder and Mathias, op cit.

that is critical to virtually every bodily system. A healthy level of vitamin D in your body can:

- ◆ *Help prevent at least 16 types of cancer*
- ◆ *Strengthen the heart and lower blood pressure*
- ◆ *Keep blood sugars steady and help prevent diabetes*
- ◆ *Minimize depression*
- ◆ *Help prevent obesity*
- ◆ *Strengthen bones and joints*
- ◆ *Reduce dental cavities by as much as 50 percent[94]*
- ◆ *Help prevent kidney disease*
- ◆ *Improve digestive health*
- ◆ *Help relieve menopausal symptoms*
- ◆ *Help prevent autoimmune diseases*
- ◆ *Lengthen life span*

CAUTION: Consult with your healthcare practitioner about healthy sun exposure, if you or your family have a history of skin cancer.

BOOSTING VITAMIN D PRODUCTION

Light-skinned people need at least 20 minutes of direct sunlight on the face, arms and legs, three times a week, or as much as an hour daily. If you are concerned about skin cancer, cover areas that are more at risk or which have received repeated sunburns.

Dark-skinned people need several times the exposure needed by light-skinned people, especially in winter and in colder climates where clothing conceals more of the skin. Dark pigments block more of the ultraviolet rays that help manufacture vitamin D.

Boston University researcher Michael Holick commented on the challenges for dark-skinned people living in colder climates, saying, "We think it's why African

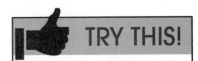

TRY THIS!

TIP: Set Your Target High
TIP is explained on page 201.

- *Tap to statements such as these: "I love being outdoors. I love the feel of sun on my skin. I love walking barefoot. I release my fear of the sun and skin cancer. I am not 'too busy' to spend time in nature. My life is energized when I spend time in nature."*

---

94   Sherry Baker, *Vitamin D Cuts Cavities in Half*, www.naturalnews.com/038183_vitamin_d_cavities_dental_health.html (January 2014).

Americans develop more prostate cancer, breast cancer and colon cancer and get more aggressive forms of those cancers." Holick, who has published hundreds of studies on vitamin D, encourages most dark-skinned people to dramatically increase their exposure to healthy sunlight.[95]

The vitamin D that is produced in the upper layers of your skin can take several hours to be absorbed into the body. Since vitamin D is water-soluble, it is best not to bathe or shower immediately after sunlight exposure. If you do bathe, use soap only on the areas of your body that do not receive sunlight, because soap is even more aggressive than water at removing vitamin D.[96]

You can boost your vitamin D input a little by consuming oily fish like salmon, cod and tuna, or by drinking milk. I do not recommend using unnatural tanning beds. The better answer is to take vitamin D3 supplements, especially in the winter.

The FDA encourages the average person to consume 200 IU of vitamin D3 daily, although other sources recommend 600 to 5,000 IUs. Higher quantities are needed for dark-skinned people year-round, as well as for everybody in the winter months. Take vitamin D with a little food containing fat, since fats aid the body in assimilating vitamin D.

I also recommend taking a 25-OH (25-hydroxy) vitamin D test about twice a year. These tests are commercially available and your test results should be from 32 to 80 mg/ml, although a higher number in that range is better.

BRING NATURE INDOORS

Bring nature into your home with houseplants, open windows and natural lighting. Use a dehumidifier, if necessary, to reduce mold and mildew – especially in crawl spaces and basements. Keep your house clean and eliminate all pet smells, hair and dander.

The Environmental Working Group has a Healthy Home Checklist which covers the following areas:[97]

◆ *Kitchen. Non-stick cookware causes toxic fumes. Glass food containers are healthier than plastic, especially if they are microwaved. Consider using a water filter, especially if you have city water. (See the Water chapter for more information.) Canned food may be unhealthy, so eat fresh or frozen.*

---

95   Kim Painter, *Your Health: Skin Color Matters in the Vitamin D Debate*, http://usatoday30.usatoday.com/news/ health/painter/2009-04-19-your-health_N.htm?csp=YahooModule_News (January 2014).

96   *Vitamin D3*, www.fda.gov/Food/IngredientsPackagingLabeling/GRAS/SCOGS/ucm261118.htm (January 2014).

97   *Your Healthy Home Checklist*, www.ewg.org/research/healthy-home-tips/tip-14-your-healthy-home-checklist (January 2014).

- **Bathroom.** *Avoid fluoridated toothpaste, anti-bacterial liquid soap and vinyl shower curtains. Consider not using hair spray, de-tanglers and body sprays. Use fragrance-free products and avoid using air fresheners, room deodorizers, unnatural cosmetics, scented candles and perfumes. Many of the chemicals used in fragrances are potential human carcinogens.*[98]
- **Laundry and Cleaning Supplies.** *Try to buy green cleaning products. Consider using natural products like vinegar, baking soda, water and plain old rags. You might not need dryer sheets, fabric softener and chlorine bleach.*
- **General.** *Try using low VOC paints, and watch out for lead paint in older homes. Foam furniture and mattresses are treated with toxic fire retardant chemicals, so cover them or get rid of them. Consider using full-spectrum lights. Avoid toxic pesticides and insecticides. Choose non-toxic toys for children.*

This basic rule of thumb could save your life: natural is always better. Nature nurtures our healthy gene expressions.

NATURE IS THE NATURAL CHOICE

As with each of the Eight Essentials, balance is the key. You obviously should not sit in the sun until your skin turns red. It's too bad we don't have an indoor indicator to let us know when to stop working under the fluorescent lights or sitting motionless in front of an electronic device. Can you imagine if our skin started to turn blue? We'd all rush like stampeding buffalo for the sunshine and open air.

Some of my best memories in life happened when I was enjoying nature, whether I was hiking with family and friends, working on the farm, going for a run on the perfect day, sweating in the hot sun or picking the ice crystals out of my beard (when I had one). Few things in life can eclipse the joys that you'll find in nature.

Tip the balance in favor of nature and sunshine today. Do not neglect the sunshine vitamin, vitamin D, and its amazing potential to boost essential phytonutrients and immunity factors. Kick off your shoes and run barefoot through the grass. Skip the excuses and – instead – skip on down the driveway. It's not too hot or too cold – not if you dress appropriately. You are not too

---

98   *The Toxic Effects of Perfume*, www.care2.com/greenliving/toxic-effects-of-perfume.html#ixzz2XSO7ZjqV (January 2014).

busy to improve your health by communing with nature. Even if you spend every waking hour in a dense urban area, you can still experience nature.

Take a walk in the park. Sunbathe on the roof or balcony. Go to the window and experience the peaceful, rejuvenating energy of simply watching an autumn leaf fall, or letting the breeze sift through your hair. Close your eyes and feel the life-giving rays of the sun warm your face. Nature is everywhere; all you have to do is reach out and touch it. You can take our free, Whole Person Appraisal at www.DrFrankKing.com to identify additional, life-affirming choices regarding nature.

Don't be like a polar bear in the desert. Allow nature to nurture you. Nature nurtures your healthy gene expressions, awakening the healing power within you. Nature can be one of your closest companions in the Healing Revolution. Take back your natural environment!

SELF-EVALUATION
NATURE

My Life-Destroying Choices
(e.g.: too much time indoors, too many excuses not to be cold, wet or uncomfortable outside)

My Life-Affirming Choices
(e.g.: eliminate my excuses for not getting outside more, find and appreciate nature in the city)

My Life-Destroying Choices	My Life-Affirming Choices
1	1
2	2
3	3
4	4
5	5
6	6
7	7

The Story of
Heart Attack Grill

A woman in her 40s collapsed unconscious while smoking a cigarette and eating a Double Bypass Burger at the Heart Attack Grill in Las Vegas, Nevada. Two months earlier, another customer had a heart attack while eating a Triple Bypass Burger. One year before that, the Heart Attack Grill's 575-pound spokesperson died at the age of 29.

The Heart Attack Grill's Quadruple Bypass Burger is built with four beef patties, lard-dipped buns, American cheese and 20 pieces of bacon. It packs more than 8,000 calories, enough to fuel the average person for four days, according to the FDA's 2000-calories-per-day guideline. That is not counting side orders of Flatliner Fries cooked in lard, butterfat shakes, beer, soft drinks and candy cigarettes for the kids.

Heart Attack Grill staff dress like nurses. They take "prescriptions" from customers who are called "patients." A bell rings to announce customers who weigh in at over 350 pounds, who then eat free. An off-service ambulance is parked in front of the establishment.

Owner Jon Basso, who dresses like a doctor, established the Heart Attack Grill with the stated intention of serving "nutritional pornography" – food "so bad for you it's shocking." Basso claims, "I have had warning labels since day one when we opened in 2005 telling people how bad our food is for you. I think that skirts any liability we might have."

Regarding the customer who hit the floor while eating the bacon-covered burger with lard-dipped buns – who was also smoking and drinking a margarita – Basso stated, "I would say the woman gave her body every single thing it could handle and it finally gave out."[99]

The restaurant's slogan is "Taste worth dying for."

Now, in case you wondered why we need a Healing Revolution ...

---

99   *Heart Attack Grill Customer Collapses While Eating Double Bypass Burger, Smoking,* www.huffingtonpost. com/2012/04/24/heart-attack-grill-collapse_n_1448694.html and Heart Attack Grill Website, www.heartattackgrill.com/ (January 2014).

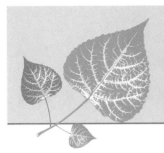

ESSENTIAL #7:
RELATIONSHIPS

True friendship is like sound health; the value of it is seldom known until it is lost.

– 18th century author
Charles Caleb Colton

When we were first married, my wife, Suzie, got together regularly with a tight band of lady friends who were all in a similar stage of life. Soon the babies started coming. That's when Suzie mentioned to the others that one of the ladies hadn't come to one of their gatherings in a couple months.

"I haven't seen her since she had her baby," Suzie said.

"Me neither," one of her friends agreed. "I left her a couple messages, but she hasn't returned my calls."

"Same with me," said another.

"My husband talked to her husband," said a third, "and he says their baby is crying all the time. She's exhausted. She needs a break."

"She needs to get out of the house."

"At least for one evening."

"We should kidnap her!"

"Yeah!"

"Let's do something fun together."

"Let's take her hostage!"

Within moments, a plot was hatched. The fearless ringleader contacted the husband to read him the terms.

"We're coming in," she informed the man. "We're getting her out, and you better be ready. We mean business, okay? Now here is what we want …"

The husband braced himself for the worst to be expected in a hostage situation.

"First of all," the woman demanded, "get her to pump breast milk in advance so you can feed the baby while we're out. Second, tell her to look good. She'll want to blow-dry her hair and put on make-up. Third, have her ready by 6 p.m. And finally, don't expect to see her again ... not for five or six hours. Understand?"

The husband was unusually cooperative. All conditions were operational when the ringleader arrived, right on schedule.

The wife emerged from her bunker looking tired and haggard, but at least her hair and make-up were up to specifications. She was led to the car and driven to the rendezvous point – a local restaurant – where she was reunited with her caring comrades.

They filled the next three hours with fun, food, love and laughter. This woman's tense shoulders relaxed, the hollow look in her eyes disappeared, her smile widened and she simply came alive.

One woman would talk about her bratty baby and another would tell a story of her colicky kid. Each story was better than the one before. Explosive diapers, breasts that leaked like faucets and mother-in-law tensions all became things to laugh about. These women were like sisters who had no inhibitions, who had never been apart.

But all too soon, it was time to go their separate ways.

"Thank you so much for this evening," the kidnapped woman said. "You have made me feel so special. I love my baby and husband so much, but after only seeing them and nobody else for such a long time, I was beginning to feel so weird. My gosh, I didn't realize how much I needed you all!"

They hugged. They laughed. They cried. They talked for another hour out in the parking lot.

Finally the woman demanded, "I have got to get home now. My boobs are about to burst! But I wouldn't trade this evening for the world. You have saved my life!"

This priceless meeting recharged and rejuvenated more than one woman that night. My wife tells me that her friend came out of her shell after that and began to intentionally get together with her friends. She just needed a little help climbing out of her trench.

RELATIONSHIPS ARE ESSENTIAL FOR LIFE

A person who is full of himself has no room for anybody else. Humans are social beings. Too many people know each other's names but not their hearts. People need people to thrive and survive. Sick relationships lead to sick bodies and minds.

> *Pleasant words are a honeycomb sweet to the soul and healing to the bones.*
>
> *– The Bible (Proverbs 16:24)*

A study of more than 309,000 people discovered that a lack of strong relationships increased the risk of premature death from any cause by a whopping 50 percent. Another study found dementia to be lowest in people 75 and over who had strong friendships.[100] Compared to married people, mortality rates are 50 percent higher for unmarried women and *250 percent higher* for unmarried men ages 45 to 65. Socially isolated people are at greater risk of depression, heart disease and early death. Happily married people are healthier and better off financially.[101]

Researchers attribute excellent health in the Italian immigrant town of Roseto, Pennsylvania, in the early 1900s, to their strong social connections. Similar studies showed excellent health among traditional Amish communities that emphasize strong relationships.[102] People in these communities value time spent together, and they make the effort to help each other through sickness and hardship.

Isolation marginalizes people. Friends, family and colleagues give perspectives that people are unable to see alone. I know this from personal experience. My trusted friends have saved me from making some really bad decisions. Once, my wife, Suzie, warned me against making a business deal that I thought was as logical and safe as it possibly could be. Suzie had no logical reason to oppose the deal, but in her gut she felt that something wasn't right. When I made the deal based on what looked to be irrefutable logic, unfortunately it went bad. To her credit, she never said a word against me. Everybody can be spared heartache if they take time to discuss important decisions with a close friend.

Listening to gut instincts should become a part of our logic. The enteric nervous system in the gut has been called the "second brain," having 100 million neurons and operating independently of the brain and central nervous system. Suzie is well-connected with her enteric nervous system.

---

100   Harvard Health, *Strong Relationships Are Good for Your Health*, www.ihavenet.com/Health-Strong-Relationships-Are-Good-For-Your-Health-Harvard-Health.html (January 2014).

101   Linda J. Waite and Maggie Gallagher, *The Case for Marriage: Why Married People Are Happier, Healthier, and Better off Financially*, www.psychpage.com/family/brwaitgalligher.html (January 2014).

102   *Human Connections and Why We Get Sick*, http://blueheronhealthnews.com/site/2013/12/24/human-connection-and-why-we-get-sick-2/; and *The Roseto Effect: a 50-year Comparison of Mortality Rates*, www.ncbi.nlm.nih.gov/pmc/articles/PMC1695733/ (January 2014).

The only bad decisions I've made are when I didn't listen to my wife's deeper instincts. Hopefully you have a trusted advisor like that, with gifted gut instincts.

English-speaking, Western people may be some of the richest and loneliest people in the world. Perhaps you have seen a tank-like SUV drive into the garage of a big suburban home, then the doors clang shut like the drawbridge on a castle. The fortress walls are impregnable so the king or queen inside will feel safe, surrounded by crown jewels and personal electronic devices. Many of these people live alone, and many don't even know their neighbors. Contrast this with a poor, tribal village in the so-called "less fortunate" parts of the world, where everybody knows everybody and where packs of little children migrate seamlessly from house to house. A friend of mine was in the Philippines and casually told a small group of people that many Americans don't know their neighbors. The Filipino people laughed, thinking my friend must be joking. Community relationships are so important to those people that they couldn't imagine anybody living without them. We may be the richest of people, but rich in what way? We are poorest in some of the things that matter most.

Western culture places such a high value on individualism – on the Lone Ranger ethic of lifting yourself up by your own boot straps – that too many people suffer and even die of sick relationships. My belief is that it takes a team to fulfill a dream. Even the Lone Ranger had Tonto.

Good relationships make us feel so good because they boost endorphins in the body. Endorphins are the feel-good hormone. Random acts of kindness create a rush of endorphins. I personally like to measure success in terms of endorphins more than with achievements or dollars. Let's strive to become endorphinaires instead of millionaires!

TOXIC RELATIONSHIPS

Unfortunately, the absolute best and worst thing that has ever happened to many people is the same: relationships.

Toxic relationships can make you sick. Negative interactions with family and friends cause bad health and reduced immunity to disease. Women in unsatisfying marital-type commitments have a higher risk of cardiovascular disease than those in satisfying relationships. "Dozens of studies have shown that people who have satisfying relationships with family, friends, and their community are happier, have fewer health problems, and live longer.

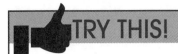
TIP: Healthy Boundaries

*Tap Into Potential (TIP)
is explained on page 201.*

*Good friends start with yourself.
Try tapping to:*

- *"I want good, healthy, happy,
life-affirming friends."*
- *"I deserve good, healthy, life-
affirming friends."*
- *"I actively seek great friends."*
- *"I cultivate purposeful
friendships."*
- *"I AM a good, happy, healthy,
life-affirming friend."*

Conversely, a relative lack of social ties is associated with depression and later-life cognitive decline, as well as with increased mortality."[103]

I knew a woman who called herself an "*[expletive]* magnet." Each man she married was more abusive and more alcoholic than the one before. Remarkably, she didn't see a pattern. Emotionally-sick people often get stuck in a revolving door of nightmares: They hook up with sick people, they get hurt bad, they run away, they hook up with sick people again, and the cycle continues. Relationships that should bring life and happiness are instead killing many people.

If you are to take back your relationships in the Healing Revolution, draw firm boundaries around your heart and your self-respect. Know how to say "no" to bad relationships. Know how to fix relationships that have positive potential. Know how to find and keep good friends, especially when it comes to healing buddies. Cultivate a positive image of yourself and how you deserve to be treated. Desire good friendships. Believe you will have good friends. Then simply become a good friend.

TO HAVE A FRIEND, BE A FRIEND

*The only way to have a
friend is to be one.*

*– Ralph Waldo
Emerson*

Good friends are worth more than gold. One fundamental principle of relational health is reciprocity, or give-and-take. In a healthy relationship, one person is not always giving and the other taking, but each person gives and receives in a balanced way. Codependent relationships, for example, are defined by one sick person and one controlling or rescuing person. Parasitic relationships

---

103   Harvard Health, *Strong Relationships Are Good for Your Health*, *www.ihavenet.com/Health-Strong-Relationships-Are-Good-For-Your-Health-Harvard-Health.html* (January 2014).

happen when one person sucks the life out of the other person. These are not healthy relationships.

Healthy people set healthy boundaries over their time, their possessions, their bodies and their lives. These healthy boundaries tell other people, even close friends and spouses, where they are not allowed to go.

Do you remember having a "conversation" with somebody who always talks, who never stops to listen? That's not the kind of a "friend" you want to be. Enter friendship with a readiness to give and take, with a good sense of balance in everything you share. This is a healthy relationship. To have a friend, be a friend.

Maybe you are the person standing all alone in a room full of strangers who says, "I don't know anybody here." Here's what I would suggest: Go talk to somebody just like you, who is standing all alone. Then you'll both know somebody and you just might make a friend for life.

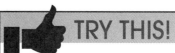

TRY THIS!

MRT and TIP:
Life-Giving Friendships
(see Essential #8 for help using MRT and TIP)

- *The following are some examples of statements you might test using MRT: "I am seeking life-giving relationships. I will find life-giving relationships. I am a good friend to others. I am a good listener. My friends like me. My friends will protect me and watch out for me. I accept myself. I accept others. I am not too critical of myself. I am not too critical of others."*
- *Use TIP with weak statements that need strengthening.*
- *Make lifestyle changes, where appropriate, to improve your life-giving friendships.*
- *Fill the holes in your wholeness with the help of our Whole Person Appraisal at www.DrFrankKing.com.*

If you want more fun, more joy, more peace, more health and more wholeness in your friendships, learn to generate these qualities from within and share them with others. Experience more feel-good endorphins by sharing time, energy and compassion with others. Become a good listener and deeply care about others. To make a friend, be a friend.

It is good and natural for you to have different levels of friendship. Casual friendships are important, but intentionally seek out deeper, brother-from-another-mother or sister-from-another-mister types of friendships. Healthy people have at least one other friend to whom they can confess their deepest needs and concerns. These friendships usually don't "just happen." A deeply-bonded relationship is a garden that needs tending and cultivation, so create good, healthy relationships.

KNOW YOURSELF

Knowing yourself is an important part of being a good friend. It helps to know how you are wired and how to re-wire yourself where necessary to prevent blowing fuses when you start to experience friction in your relationships. For example, if you are a talkative extrovert who hates silence as much as nature abhors a vacuum, think twice before becoming soul mates with someone who needs plenty of quiet time to recharge.

You also may or may not be aware of unresolved emotional issues stemming from past negative experiences in your life. While this is the subject of entire books, these issues can sabotage you and your relationships if you leave them unchecked. Work through these issues with someone whom you trust. Use MRT and TIP. Try using my free, Whole Person Appraisal at www.DrFrankKing.com to get to know yourself, create your picture of wholeness and identify a plan for reaching that place.

I also advise people not to rush quickly into a marital-type, physical relationship. All the "trouble" of dating slowly and getting to know a person well before giving them everything you have is much less bothersome than the crushing heartache of a bad split.

You have perhaps heard of several tests that help you identify your personality type. I have found the DISC profile test to be a terrific tool. DISC stands for four primary personality types: Dominant, Influential, Steady and Compliant. Your personality will likely be a blend of two categories, and the DISC test shows what tendencies are indicative of each type. The four categories are:

► *Dominance: Direct, decisive, independent and to the point. Bottom line and results oriented. Strong-willed, enjoy challenges and look for immediate results.*
► *Influence: Optimistic, social and outgoing. Enjoy being on teams, sharing openly, entertaining and motivating others.*
► *Steadiness: Team players, cooperative and supportive of others. Prefer being in the background, working in a stable environment. Often good listeners, preferring to avoid conflict and change.*
► *Compliance: Cautious and concerned. Focused on what is "correct," quality and details. Planning ahead and concerned about accuracy.*

The DISC test gives guidance about how different personality types work together, warning of potentially caustic communication and interactions. Still, we are most fulfilled when we have relationships with all different types of people. None of these traits are better or worse than the others. The key is to know your own strengths and weaknesses, and to understand and respect the dominant traits in the people you know and work with most closely.

Knowing personality types can help you maximize your friendships. It can also tell you what types of physical ailments you might be susceptible to. A free, basic DISC profile test is available online at: www.123test.com/disc-personality-test/index.php.

Tips for Great Friendships

▷ *Take the first step toward making a friend, if necessary*
▷ *Change yourself, not others*
▷ *Practice grace*
▷ *Give and take*
▷ *Respect others*
▷ *Respect yourself and maintain boundaries*
▷ *Develop relationships that relate in all areas of life including work, hobbies, family, fitness, faith, healing and personal interests.*

MARRIAGE, FAMILY, SEX

Every time I come home, I have a smile on my face … and I'm met by two excitedly wagging tails. Our two dogs run and yelp to announce my arrival. They jump up on my legs and beg for attention, looking like the happiest creatures on earth. Sometimes, my wife, Suzie, in her cute way will come trotting and wagging up to me, mimicking the dogs as she jumps and paws for attention. She proves that this principle works: If you want more attention, be more attentive.

In the grand design of things, marriage and family is the first place to build healthy relationships. As mentioned earlier, research shows that married people live longer, are physically and mentally healthier, are happier, recover from illness faster, and are financially better-off than singles. Undoubtedly these benefits spill over to their children. A healthy, lifelong, marital-like commitment builds trust, selfless love and holistic health in a way that is difficult to find elsewhere.

Social scientist Dr. Arthur Brooks examined vast amounts of empirical data to determine that, "42 percent of married Americans said they were very happy. Only 23 percent of never-married people said this, as well as 20 percent of those who were widowed, 17 percent of divorced people and 11 percent of those who were separated (but not divorced) from their spouses."[104]

The reality is that divorce happens. I know, because it happened to me. A person is not bad because a marriage turns bad. My father used to say, "If you fall, fall forward. That way you'll be ahead when you get up." So the important thing is to get back up if your marriage fails and make things better for yourself and especially for your kids (if you have any). This, however, is a topic for another book.

Let's talk about sex. Sex is an amazing, wonderful part of the Healing Revolution. Sex can and should be mutually beneficial, fun and fulfilling for couples, for many years longer than conventional wisdom might tell you – without the aid of drugs that don't address the causes of dysfunction and have long lists of scary side effects.

The act of giving your greatest intimacy to your partner is an act that binds you to that person like nothing else can do. It is not healthy to make and break those intimate connections that are deeper and more spiritual than modern science can yet quantify. Research shows that married people have sex more often than couples who live together, and say it is more fulfilling.[105]

I have treated sexual dysfunction for many years. A healthy balance of proper exercise, diet, relationships, sleep and all Eight Essentials can help improve sex. Tap Into Potential (TIP) is a wonderful tool for refocusing sexual urges to where they ought to be. My website, www.DrFrankKing.com, has a free Whole Person Appraisal that can help you identify other possible causes and solutions for sexual dysfunction.

> *Oh the comfort, the inexpressible comfort of feeling safe with a person; having neither to weigh thoughts nor measure words, but to pour them all out, just as they are, chaff and grain together, knowing that a faithful hand will take and sift them, keep what is worth keeping, and then, with a breath of kindness, blow the rest away.*
>
> **– English author Dinah Maria Mulock Craik**

---

104   Arthur Brooks, *Gross National Happiness* (New York: Basic Books, 2008).

105   Linda J. Waite and Maggie Gallagher, *The Case for Marriage: Why Married People Are Happier, Healthier, and Better off Financially*, www.psychpage.com/family/brwaitgalligher.html (January 2014).

TIP: For a Better Marriage

Tap Into Potential (TIP)
is explained on page 201.

- *Sooner or later every marital-type relationship will go through challenges.*
- *Use TIP to get the positive spark going again. Try tapping to phrases like the following: "My spouse is beautiful/handsome. I want to spend more quality time with him/her. I am seeing more of his/her good qualities and less of the bad. I get excited about my partner. When I am attracted to other people, I am reminded of my spouse. I am discovering new surprises, new gifts, new ways to make my partner happy. I like my spouse. I love my spouse. I adore my spouse."*

TAKE THIS JOB AND LOVE IT

Johnny Paycheck sang "Take this job and shove it," but in the Healing Revolution I hear people saying, "Take this job and *love* it!"

Unfortunately, the Gallup Poll organization found that a whopping 71 percent of Americans are disengaged at work, meaning they dislike or hate their jobs.[106] Moreover, those who hate their jobs are at higher risk of mental disorders, high blood pressure, heart disease[107], and they are more likely to smoke. [108]

Make a quick list of how many waking hours you spend each week at all your activities, and if you are like the average person, you will discover that "work" is at the top of the list. You will spend more time working than you will commuting, exercising, eating, doing chores, recreating, interacting with friends or family, or possibly the sum of all your waking-hour activities combined.

Given the fact that you spend so much of your life at work, don't you want to make your job as positive of an experience as possible? Most people spend more time with co-workers than they do with their family. Grow healthy roots with co-workers and you will bear greater fruits. Cultivate a positive attitude by working gratefully, not grudgingly. Get a reputation for not taking part in those grumbling and back-biting sessions. If you are being

---

106   *Majority of American Workers Not Engaged in Their Jobs*, www.gallup.com/poll/150383/majority-american-workers-not-engaged-jobs.aspx (January 2014).

107   *Hating Your Job is as Bad for your Health as Being Unemployed, Research Warns*, www.dailymail.co.uk/health/article-2237371/Hating-job-bad-health-unemployed-researchers-warn.html (January 2014).

108   *Americans Who Hate Their Jobs are More Likely to Smoke*, www.gallup.com/poll/164162/americans-hate-jobs-likely-smoke.aspx (January 2014).

suffocated in an environment that makes it impossible for you to breathe freely with new life and joy each day, consider finding a new job. But while you are in that difficult position, make the best of this opportunity to nurture an attitude that is better, not bitter.

Stop and consider if you are part of the problem or the solution. Try using TIP to realign your mind with life-giving attitudes at work. Be the change that you hope to see.

HELPING OTHERS

> To keep the body in good health is a duty, otherwise we shall not be able to keep our mind strong and clear.
>
> — Gautama the Buddha

Research shows that helping others is good for mental and physical health. It helps fight depression and aids in recovery from illness. It's a powerful means of staving off depression in older people whose life partners have died. Volunteerism lengthens lifespan and reduces the risk of disability. People who volunteer with two or more organizations for 100 hours a year or more get the biggest rewards. But even those who volunteer for less than two hours a week live healthier and longer.[109] One study found that retirees who helped others with transportation, errands, shopping, housework, childcare or other tasks were half as likely to die over a five year period as those who didn't volunteer.[110]

Consider performing random acts of kindness: Give a gift to a homeless person or fix your neighbor's broken whatever. Volunteer at an animal shelter or nursing home. The possibilities are endless – and so is the payback.

With your growing knowledge of health, one of the best ways to help others is with their health. Be a healing buddy! So many ailments are unnecessary. Imagine the rich rewards you will receive when you help others find health and wholeness. This is the Healing Revolution solution!

---

109   *The Health Benefits of Volunteering: A Review of Recent Research*, www.nationalservice.gov/sites/default/files/documents/07_0506_hbr_brief.pdf (January 2014).
110   *19 Healthy Reasons to Help Others*, www.huffingtonpost.com/2011/07/28/health-benefits-of-volunteering-helping-others_n_909713.html#s316118title=Helpers_Live_Longer (January 2014).

FURRY FRIENDS

Pets are good for your health. They lessen anxiety, boost immunity and lower risk of allergies and asthma.[111] Just having a pet in your lap can lower your blood pressure. Plus, they are great listeners and they give unconditional love.[112]

I have seen how pets can be healing agents in the home. My wife's mom who had Parkinson's disease lost her very special cat, Shakori, when somebody let him out the back door. Suzie's mom was sure that Shakori had been hit by a car. The family members checked every animal shelter around, but they couldn't find the poor animal. Suzie's mom's health took a dive over the next few weeks. She'd been an avid reader all her life, but she lost the ability to read and concentrate. Finally Suzie's brother happened to stop at a shelter about 45 minutes away and they were shocked to find Shakori there, six months after he had disappeared! You should have seen how Suzie's mom perked up when Shakori came home and cuddled in her lap. She was soon able to focus and read again. And she got so protective of that cat.

"Shut the door!" she would always yell whenever anybody came or went.

That animal was at least partially instrumental in restoring my mother-in-law's health. I've heard many other similar stories of companion animals that have worked nothing short of miracles in people's lives. We are intimately interconnected with everything in our environment, including our pets, farm animals, birds, gardens and so much more.

Animal companions are good for health and wholeness. Maybe you want to thank your pet for being one of your healing buddies in the Healing Revolution.

---

111   While pets lower the *risk* of asthma, they may exacerbate lung conditions that already exist.

112   *5 Ways Pets can Improve your Health,* www.webmd.com/hypertension-high-blood-pressure/features/health-benefits-of-pets (January 2014).

HEALING HAPPENS
WHEN PEOPLE GET TOGETHER

> *The greatest good you can do for another is not just to share your riches but to reveal to him his own.*
>
> *– 19th century British Prime Minister Benjamin Disraeli*

More times than I can recall, I have been on an airplane, at a party or at an informal gathering when someone tells me about an ache, pain or health issue. It could be anything from a sore muscle to heartburn. Often I tell them I'm a naturopath and a chiropractor, and I ask if they want some help with their condition. Nearly every time, their answer is a resounding, "Yes!" Suzie and I are always prepared to give them a simple homeopathic remedy, or show them one of the Hands On Techniques, as explained in the next chapter. The vast majority of people we meet experience immediate, positive results. Before I know it, three or four others are lined up to share the healing joy.

As mentioned early in this book, participants of the Daniel Plan weight loss program lost twice as much weight if they partnered with other people in the program. Friendships are key to success. It's beneficial for everybody, as each one gives and each one receives. That's the beauty of the Healing Revolution. The gift of health keeps on giving.

I have a vision of people in the Healing Revolution who rise up like an army of grassroots healers, offering safe, natural help and healing for the masses. I have a vision of Healing Parties – whether spontaneous or organized – where people use MRT and TIP ... where we offer commonsense safe, natural help and advice to each other ... where we share healthy foods and recipes ... where we walk, bike, do Energizing Techniques (ETs) and Hands On Techniques (HOTs) together. Perhaps I am describing what you and your Healing Buddies are already doing.

Community may not be a high value in this me-centered, individualistic culture, but it is for the Healing Revolution. Take back the power and potential of relationships!

You can find more of my free articles and videos at www.DrFrankKing. com. Feel free to share that website with the people you meet who are in need of a Healing Revolution.

SELF-EVALUATION
RELATIONSHIPS

My Life-Destroying Choices
*(e.g.: not making time for
relationships, not maintaining
boundaries to protect myself)*

My Life-Affirming Choices
*(e.g.: seek deeper, stronger, more
healthy relationships; stop doing
everything alone)*

1

1

2

2

3

3

4

4

5

5

6

6

7

7

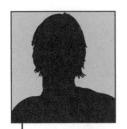

Breanna's Story:
The Doubting Spouse

Bill wasn't sick a day in his life. Breanna, on the other hand, barely found the energy to get out of bed each morning.

Strangely, it should have been the other way around. Breanna ate a strict vegetarian diet. She tried to stay fit and use natural products in the home. Her husband Bill, on the other hand, was religious about eating meat, donuts and sweets. He was active in athletics, but only as far as armchair sports go.

Breanna came into my clinic for help with headaches, fatigue and severe PMS. As I got to know Brenna over the next few visits, and as she began to see improvements in her health, she couldn't help but say a few words about her husband Bill's attitudes toward natural health.

"He's not into all this 'natural crap,' as he calls it. He thinks you natural doctors are a bunch of kooks. Then he rubs it in by reminding me that he's never been sick a day in his life, while he's breaking all the rules as far as health goes."

I'd known other people like Bill who had strong constitutions – the constitution of a cockroach, I call it – strong enough to sustain their bad habits for years until the floor caves in.

"I'd love to meet him," I said. "It may sound strange, but he's my kind of guy. I have always enjoyed talking with people who think I'm crazy!"

Actually I've rarely had a meeting with someone like Bill that didn't turn out great for everyone involved. The next time Breanna came for a visit, Bill accompanied her with his hands in his pockets and a gruff look on his face.

"Dr. King," said Breanna, "this is my husband Bill."

"Glad to meet you, Bill," I said.

Bill reluctantly shook my hand, then stood bolt-upright with his arms crossed.

"I was telling Bill about how much better I feel since I came to you. He was actually shocked when I told him you convinced me to stop being a vegetarian!"

Breanna laughed. Bill looked as cold as a character from Mount Rushmore.

"We did some tests," I explained, "and learned that Breanna was deficient in some of the nutrients that come from healthy meat. A vegetarian diet isn't suitable for her constitutional make-up. That's why she was feeling so tired all the time."

"That's right," affirmed Breanna.

"The same thing happened to me when I was on a vegetarian diet for several years," I added.

Breanna and I exchanged nervous grins. Bill just stood there.

"So Bill," I said, hoping for a warming of the weather, "is there anything I can do for you today? I won't charge you a thing for our first consultation. Breanna says you're a healthy guy, but everyone has something they'd like help with. How about you?"

Bill looked to the floor for a moment, then turned his eyes to the ceiling.

"My hands," is all he said.

I could see that the skin on his hands was cracked, seeping, red and swollen.

"He's an auto mechanic," Breanna explained, "and he always comes home smelling like grease and gasoline."

"But I don't want any of that yoga, stand-on-your-head, poke-me-with-needles crap," Bill added.

I learned that Bill spent much of the day with his hands in a smorgasbord of petrochemical toxins.

"You can start by wearing latex gloves," I said, "Your body is absorbing those chemicals right through your skin. I'll also give you some homeopathic remedies to detoxify your body and heal your cracked skin. What's more, I'd like to give you a list of antioxidant foods that will help you naturally detoxify."

I took a few minutes to explain the negative effects of those harmful chemicals on his body. He took my advice. When I saw him a week or two later, his hands were doing much better.

Encouraged by these results, I asked Bill if there was anything else I could help him with.

Bill thought a moment, then said, "Energy, I suppose. Maybe it's just 'cause I get up early each morning and work hard all day. Probably can't help that."

After probing a little deeper, I learned about his lifestyle habits, including his morning, noon and afternoon visits to the vending machine for chemically-enhanced, refinery-sweetened, so-called "food" products. I gave him suggestions for a few healthy food alternatives that he was willing to try.

In two weeks, Bill was much more friendly. He felt better and his home life had improved. Like so many other people I have known through the years, Bill had changed from skeptic to believer. In time, he even began to refer other patients to our clinic.

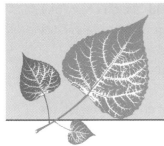

ESSENTIAL #8:
HANDS ON TECHNIQUES (HOT)

It is confidence in our bodies, minds and spirits that allows us to keep looking for new adventures, new directions to grow in, and new lessons to learn, which is what life is all about.

**– Oprah Winfrey,
"Oprah Magazine," May 2004**

Years ago, I was excited to meet my wife Suzie's family for the first time, but I had no idea that that first meeting would turn into a healing party.

Imagine Suzie at her parents' house with her brother, sister, niece, nephew and father all sprawled out on the living room floor. They were all resting comfortably after implementing some simple healing techniques, although that's probably not what it looked like to a skeptic like Suzie's mother who just entered the room.

Suzie's mom was a registered nurse practitioner, steeped in the creeds of conventional medicine. She had a look on her face as if to say, "You people have a third arm growing out of the middle of your foreheads!"

Suzie's father looked up from the floor. "Hey Norma," he said, "lie down on the floor with us. Frank just worked on me and I feel great! You're gonna love this. He really knows what he's doing."

After a little more coaxing, Norma got down on the floor. I was especially sensitive with Suzie's mom, wanting to make a positive impression on her. I used gentle pressure points on the muscles between the vertebrae of her spine to relieve tension. I also did Muscle Response Tests to identify homeopathic remedies to relieve her joint pain.

"Try some of this arthritis remedy before you go to bed tonight," I suggested, giving her a bottle of homeopathic medicine.

Reluctantly Suzie's mom used the remedy. The next morning she walked into the room looking like a million bucks.

"I never slept so good in all my life," Norma said. "I didn't have any pain whatsoever! Of course, it wasn't the adjustment or that natural medicine stuff you gave me, Frank. It was just a weird fluke."

She thought for a moment, then smiled and nodded her head. "I guess I slept so well because I'm so happy to see you all."

I'm not known for lacking words, but this brief presentation left me totally speechless.

Suzie's nephew was the only one who could manage a come-back. "But Grandma, you said you wanted help sleeping better, and ... and look what happened!"

"No, no," Norma insisted. "It's just so special to have my family here together. Still, Frank ... would you mind leaving me a bottle of that arthritis formula? ... not that I plan to use it regularly, of course."

HEALING PARTIES HAPPEN

Those kinds of healing parties happen to me all the time: in our living room, at the office, on a plane or at the beach. And they can happen to you too. All you need to get started is the heart of a healer and some of these basic Hands On Techniques. How often have you been chatting with someone at the park, the mall or while traveling and you find out they have an ache, a pain or a special health need? That's an open door to sensitively share some aspect of the Healing Revolution.

> *So long as we are in conflict with our body, we cannot find peace of mind.*
>
> **– Yoga master Georg Feuerstein**

You don't have to be an expert to help people. You only need a compassionate heart and a desire to help others. You can share this book with them. I don't know anybody who will turn down a chance to feel better.

As suggested earlier, get together with healing buddies who share your passion for health, healing and wholeness. The benefits multiply many times over when people get together for encouragement and support. Most people's instincts will naturally draw them toward the magnetism of these healing moments.

HANDS ON TECHNIQUES (HOTs)

We all need touch. Infants raised without skin-to-skin touch experience delayed development, failure to thrive and worse, death. Our vital need for touch does not go away as we mature. In this section, I am excited to share the art and science of applied therapeutic touch. These amazing techniques that I have shared with my patients for nearly four decades can take you, your family, the community and the world to higher levels of health, wholeness and happiness.

These Hands On Techniques (HOTs) can empower you in ways you never thought possible, as you make the commitment to nurture and develop them like a beautiful garden. Have a positive healing attitude and expect terrific results as you put them into practice. Imagine your health as it might be, as it should be, as it WILL be. Your attitude will determine your altitude, so fly high!

You can do some of these HOTs on yourself, while others will require the assistance of a healing buddy. I am passionate about these life-changing techniques that have proven themselves with the test of time, having safely and effectively enabled my patients to achieve greater health and happiness since the 1970s. Before you begin, however, I encourage you to take our Whole Person Appraisal at www.DrFrankKing.com. This free tool is like a snapshot, showing you the "big picture" of your health, leading you to focus on the specific areas that are most in need of wholeness. You will also find helpful videos of these and more Hands On Techniques at that website. And it's all free!

We will begin with the Muscle Response Test (MRT) and Tap Into Potential (TIP), two of the most valuable tools in the Healing Revolution.

HOT #1: MUSCLE RESPONSE TEST (MRT)[113]

▶ Communicating with your body's inner wisdom.

The Muscle Response Test (MRT) works like a truth detector to help you discover and discern what may be helpful or harmful for your life and health. You will need a healing buddy to perform MRT. Here's how it works:

---

113   This chapter explains how to do MRT. For why and for more background information, see "The Healing Revolution Explained" chapter.

MRT: The Basics

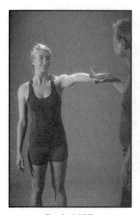

Basic MRT: Strong Response

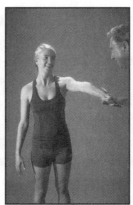

Basic MRT: Weak Response

◆ *Stand facing your healing buddy. Raise your dominant arm straight in front of you at shoulder height, parallel to the floor, with your elbow locked straight. Your partner will apply downward pressure to your wrist.*

◆ *If your arm remains firm and steady, not going down at all, that is a **strong response**.*

Next, hold some food or a household item, or make a statement related to your health. Your arm will go weak when you hold or say things that are unhealthy for you.

◆ *If your arm is weak or mushy and goes down a few inches, that is a weak response. Your healing buddy should not push down more than about three inches if you have a **weak response**.[114] Next, hold a food or household item, or make a statement related to your health. Your weak arm will go strong when you hold or say things that are healthy for you.*

Examples of Basic MRT

First, do the test (above) to see if your basic response is strong or weak. Then, hold an item (e.g., from your refrigerator, or from your cleaning supplies) and have your healing buddy test you with MRT:

▷ *If your basic response was strong, your arm will go weak if that item is not good for you.*
▷ *If your basic response was weak, your arm will go strong if that item is healthy for you.*
▷ *Similarly, you can test the truth of statements with MRT. For example, "I am getting enough sleep," "I love to make healthy choices," or "I need more vitamin D."*

---

114   A weak muscle response does not mean you are a weak person! It is simply the method your nerve is using to communicate a specific message to your muscles.

▶ MRT: Advanced

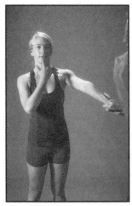

Advanced MRT

If you had a <u>strong response</u> in the basic technique (above)...

◆ *Have your healing buddy retest you while you place your other hand on a key point on your body such as your forehead, your throat (thyroid), the base of the manubrium (the bony groove at the upper edge of your breastbone), the solar plexus (where the stomach meets the lower edge of the sternum), the belly button or another point down the center line of your body. Find one point that causes MRT weakness. (Some people find that wetting their fingers with water makes it easier to obtain the necessary results.)*

◆ *While keeping your hand over the key point that causes weakness, place an item that you would like to test in your lap or under your arm, or make a statement related to your health, while your healing buddy tests you with MRT. If that item or statement is healthy for you, your arm will go strong. If that item or statement is neutral or bad for you, your arm will remain weak.*

If you had a <u>weak response</u> in the basic technique (above)...

◆ *Have your healing buddy retest you while you place your other hand on a key point on your body such as your forehead, your throat (thyroid), the base of the manubrium (the bony groove at the upper edge of your breastbone), the solar plexus (where the stomach meets the lower edge of the sternum), the belly button or another point down the center line of your body. Find one point that causes MRT strength. (Some people find that wetting their fingers with water makes it easier to obtain the necessary results.)*

◆ *While keeping your hand over the key point that causes strength, place an item that you would like to test in your lap or under your arm, or make a statement related to your health, while your healing buddy tests you with MRT. If that item or statement is unhealthy for you, your arm will go weak. If that item or statement is neutral or good for you, your arm will remain strong.*

▶ MRT: General Information

◆ Perform MRT on arms, hands, wrists and shoulders that are free from injury.

◆ Consistency is important: Your healing buddy should push with the same strength throughout MRT.

◆ Wait 5 to 7 seconds before each MRT test.

◆ A measurable energy field radiates out from every living thing. Your energy field intersects with things that you hold. For this reason, you need not be in physical contact with substances that are in packaging to test them. Simply hold the packaged item in your hand, lap, or under an arm, and MRT will be accurate. Try it and see how well it works!

◆ MRT is like any art. The more clear and focused you are, the more clear and focused will be the results. MRT has led many of my patients to insights that modern lab tests and science could not reveal. A confident, positive attitude that seeks truth will compensate for minor inconsistencies in the test procedure.

◆ If you are having trouble with MRT, try drinking a half glass of water. Dehydration can interfere with the MRT process.

Some Examples of Advanced MRT

▷ If your arm was strong in the basic test (above), hold one hand over a key point on your body that makes your arm go weak. (See text for more information.) Then place a food item in your lap or say something like, "I need more vitamin C." When your healing buddy tests you with MRT, your arm will go strong if that item or statement is healthy for you. Your arm will remain weak if the item or statement is neutral or bad for you.

▷ If your arm was weak in the basic test (above), hold one hand over a key point on your body that makes your arm go strong. Then place an item in your lap or under your arm, or say something like, "I want to exercise." When your healing buddy tests you with MRT, your arm will go weak if that item or statement is unhealthy for you. Your arm will remain strong if the item or statement is neutral or good for you.

MRT can be fun for the whole family. You'll share lots of laughs with your kids while finding healthy and tasty alternatives for all the fake foods and ill thrills of the 21st century. More and more people are discovering the powerful potential of MRT – from professional medical doctors to ordinary men, women and children who are struggling to make sense of the barrage of questionable health choices today.

This is merely an introduction to a complex topic that can help guide all your lifestyle choices as they apply to the Eight Essentials. For helpful videos and articles about MRT, visit www.DrFrankKing.com.

HOT #2: TAP INTO POTENTIAL (TIP)

Programming for the perfect life.
"Specializing in Difficult Cases." That was the tag line for our practice. MRT and TIP were the two main reasons we were able to succeed where so many others failed.

Tap Into Potential (TIP) is a powerful tool for *change* ... for improving health and for reprogramming negative attitudes and habits to become positive ones. See "The Healing Revolution Explained" chapter for WHY you need TIP. This explains HOW to do it.

TIP is not a magic formula that will fail if your mind wanders, if your motives are impure, or if you are guilt-ridden because of past failures. Put your mind at ease and simply enjoy the process. The greater your

WHAT'S SO GREAT ABOUT THE MUSCLE RESPONSE TEST?

I love watching people's faces light up when they suddenly grasp the power of MRT. "Wow!" they say. "There is nothing I can't do with MRT! I can test all the foods in my kitchen, all my cleaning supplies, everything in my medicine chest, all my pets, my work space, my sleep space, my habits, my attitudes, my actions ... the possibilities are endless!"

That is completely true. Life is filled with choices, many of which enable you to live long and well. Misplaced steps, however, lead to a minefield of toxic consequences. MRT gives you a wealth of knowledge that may otherwise be inaccessible. This tool has the potential to take you light years ahead of where conventional medical tests today can lead you. That is why I am so excited to share this powerful HOT tool with my Healing Revolution friends!

investment, the greater your results will be. The more you tap, the more comfortable you will become. At first, the mechanics of tapping may take your full attention, but soon the physical procedure will become natural and "automatic" as you focus on what really matters.

What matters most? Remember the three powerful words to transform:

Desire.
Believe.
Become.

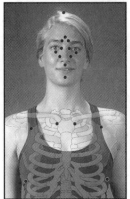

Key Tapping Points for activating health and wholeness

Begin by naming the problem (the sickness, the addiction or the attitude). Then replace that with the *new you that you want to become*. Think more about abundant health and powerful potentials than about problems. Over time, the more you tap, the more you will desire, believe and become the new, whole you.

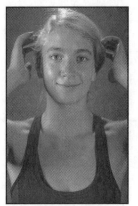

Tapping: Temple

Let each statement you make take you farther from the sickness or dysfunction and closer to health and wholeness. Keep moving forward and never look back. Learn to integrate all your senses in the process: your sight, smell, hearing, words, touch, emotions, visualizations, hopes and faith. Put your whole self into it.

Improvise freely, refining the beautiful picture of who you are becoming. Use this technique to address physical illness, emotions, pain, choices, relationships and attitudes. Use it to reduce fears, to increase performance or to prepare you to make better choices about anything. Science may not be able to fully explain how tapping translates to positive results, but the evidence in favor of TIP is overwhelming. You become what you believe and desire, in the measure to which you invest yourself in the process.

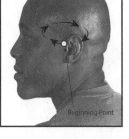

Tap in an oval around your temples

Here's how to do TIP: tap with your fingertips (as many as comfortably fit) over key acupuncture meridian points while making positive statements (verbally and in your thoughts). The most effective tapping points, using two hands at once, include:

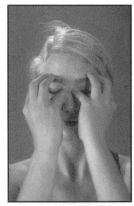

- *The temple region of the head, slightly in front and above the front edge of the ears. Tap in an oval around the temples for about five rotations while making positive statements. Tapping here first will open your filters and help your body and mind become more receptive to positive change.*

Tapping: Eyes

- *The top-center of your head, on the front portion of the "soft spot" depression (from when you were a baby).*[115]

- *Around both eyes. Your fingers will simultaneously tap near the inner corners, along your eyebrow and on the outside corner of your eyes. Your thumb will tap the middle-center below your eye. Alternately, you may tap each of these points individually.*

- *Above and below your lips, at the inner-most indentation.*

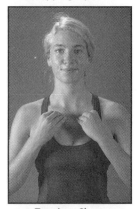

- *On each side of the top of your chest bone, below the bony protrusion where your clavicles meet your sternum.*

Tapping: Chest

Begin tapping in the temple region while making positive affirmations. Proceed from one position to the next, taking as much time as you like in each area. You may also tap with each hand simultaneously in different locations.

For example, you might make the following statements to address a bad habit or negative thought while tapping:

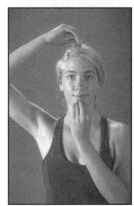

- *"From now on, I will exchange _____ (e.g., "my cravings for sweets") for healthy choices*

Tapping: Different Locations

---

115   This is the GV20 acupuncture point.

like_____ (e.g., "whole foods"). I am trading my bad desires for good ones. I am losing my bad desires and habits. Those bad desires and habits have NO power over me. I am happy and healthy with my new choice (e.g., "eating real, healthy, whole foods and becoming more whole"). This is the new, beautiful me. I am already receiving the wonderful benefits of my good choices."

New personal, relevant thoughts will come to you as you tap. Doors of new insight will open, revealing deeper revelations into yourself. Allow your new creative thoughts to take you as far as you want to go. Spend as much time on TIP as you like — sessions can vary from three to 30 minutes, as often as you choose. Use MRT, if desired, to assure yourself that positive changes are taking place before and after tapping. You can also use MRT to locate the most effective tapping points.

HOT #3: SHRINK YOUR STOMACH TECHNIQUE

The stomach size of most people in our culture has been expanded by too many years of overeating. Stretched-out stomachs contribute to greater

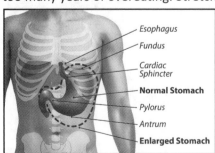

Esophagus
Fundus
Cardiac Sphincter
Normal Stomach
Pylorus
Antrum
Enlarged Stomach

hunger and food consumption. Eating junk food only makes you hungrier, since the empty calories leave your body craving the missing essential nutrients. Thankfully, this HOT technique has helped many of my patients get a grip on their appetites.

- *Eat a light meal in the evening.*
- *First thing when you get up the next morning, use the toilet to empty your bladder. Then drink 4 to 6 ounces of water.*
- *Lie on your back. Place both hands over the left side of your lower rib cage, from your lower breastbone to the front angle of your rib cage. Press firmly down and in toward the center of your stomach with your hands.*
- *Hold for about 30 seconds. You will likely hear a gurgling sound. Repeat several times, pressing your lower breastbone, ribs and the upper part of your stomach down toward the middle, until you hear no more gurgling sounds.*

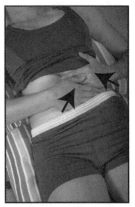

One of the Ways to
Shrink Your Stomach

- *Next, press the fingertips of both hands into the lower left side of your belly, just above your left hip bone (pulling the lower part of your stomach up toward the middle), while pressing your thumbs into your belly along the bottom of the ribs (pulling the upper part of your stomach down toward the middle).*
- *Press firmly into your gut, squeezing your thumbs and fingers together, scrunching your stomach organ into a smaller area. Hold for about 30 seconds. It is natural to hear your stomach gurgle as it shrinks.*
- *Relax. Repeat several times, until you hear no more gurgling sounds.*
- *Scrunch your stomach together from both sides, pushing toward the middle. Hold for about 30 seconds. Repeat until you hear no more gurgling sounds.*
- *Eat light meals and chew your food more times than usual, to aid in digestion and to increase feelings of being full. If you overeat, repeat this HOT technique.*
- *Repeat every morning for three days or as needed to reduce appetite and stomach size.*

WHAT'S SO WONDERFUL ABOUT the SHRINK YOUR STOMACH TECHNIQUE?

People often go to great trouble and expense, jumping through dietary hoops, in a futile attempt to curb appetite. Why not try the obvious first? A large stomach has a large appetite. It cries relentlessly for food. I have seen so many people control their hunger, take off extra pounds, improve digestion, become more satisfied with smaller portions and end recurring struggles with their weight by simply and naturally shrinking their stomach size.

Control hunger and give your body what it truly needs by eating whole foods, taking whole food supplements, using TIP and drinking plenty of pure water between meals.

HOT #4: FULL DIAPHRAGM BREATHING AND STRAPPING TECHNIQUE

The diaphragm is a reservoir of energy for a healthy body and mind. It is also the great mimicker: Diaphragm dysfunction can precipitate a wide variety of symptoms, from headaches and heartburn to hiccups and hemorrhoids.

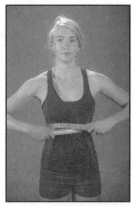

Strapping

This HOT helps expand upon the full breathing movements described in the Fitness Essential chapter (page 101), to maximize the natural, cleansing and healing powers of "vitamin O" – oxygen. Full diaphragm breathing draws air into the lower third of your lungs, which does not get used with shallow breathing.

◆ *Lie on your back and place one hand on your belly and one on your chest.*
◆ *Breathe naturally. Concentrate on your belly, which should rise with each breath in, and fall with each breath out. Your sides and lower ribs should also expand as you breathe in. These are signs that you are restoring your full, diaphragm-breathing function.*
◆ *Wrap a wide belt or strap around your lower rib cage, crossing at the bottom of your sternum. Hold it snug with your hands. (You may do this technique either standing or lying down.)*
◆ *Breathe deep while expanding your belly and lower rib cage against the belt's tension. Barely allow the belt to release against the diaphragm and rib cage's expanding movement.*
◆ ***DO NOT pull so tight with the strap as to cause pain.***
◆ *Exhale while pulling the strap tighter.*
◆ *Repeat three times, then remove the strap. You should feel more freedom and expansion in the belly, diaphragm muscle and lower rib cage while drawing more air into your lungs.*
◆ *Alternately, you may bring the belt slightly up or down. Repeat the technique to increase your breathing capacity.*

- *Be conscious of your breathing all day long. Most people need reminders (such as notes that say "Breathe!" or an automatic timer message) until the new full-breathing habit is established.*

Here's a simple test for diaphragm weakness or dysfunction: interrupt your breathing for 10 seconds – without taking a big breath first – and have your healing buddy test you with MRT. Your arm will remain strong if your diaphragm is healthy.

You can find more helpful information and my videos about this and other HOTs at www.DrFrankKing.com.

HOT #5:STRESS RECEPTOR MASSAGE TECHNIQUE

"Stress receptors" are like neurological fuses embedded in the skin that correspond to specific internal organs, muscles and body functions. Briskly massage the head's stress receptors to help reset the healthy control networks of physiologically stressed areas throughout your entire body. A time-saving alternative is to massage your face and scalp while applying shampoo or conditioner in the shower – and you won't mess up your hair! Here's how to do it:

WHAT'S SO IMPORTANT ABOUT the DIAPHRAGM BREATHING and STRAPPING TECHNIQUE?

I tested all my patient's breathing when they first came into our practice, and learned that 80 percent of them were inhaling at just 60 to 70 percent of capacity. That almost takes *my* breath away, thinking of all the priceless benefits of "Vitamin O" (oxygen) that they were missing.

Breath is life! Oxygen is the essential catalyst to all healing, and "healing" is the first word in the Healing Revolution. See how important Vitamin O is? If you are like the average person – especially if you sit scrunched up in a chair for much of the day – be as intentional as I was when I first learned to breathe years ago. I put stickers and signs on the mirrors, fridge, walls and furniture of my house that simply said, "Breathe." Try it and see how much more energy you get in return, since lack of oxygen is a primary cause of fatigue. Oxygen is readily available for everyone, and it's absolutely free!

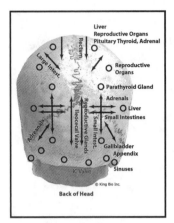

Stress Receptors:
Back of Head. Massage from the back of the head along these lines.

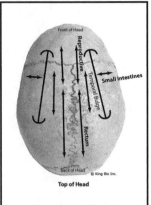

Stress Receptors:
Top of Head. Massage toward the front of the head along these lines.

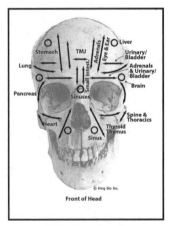

Stress Receptors:
Side of Face. Massage down toward the jaw, then horizontally to the sides.

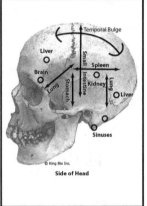

Stress Receptors:
Side of Head. Massage horizontally, vertically and in small circles.

- Relax, breathing deep and slow through your nose. Briskly massage back and forth over as large of an area of stress receptor points as your fingers and hands can cover, for about three breaths, in and out.

- Working the fingers and hands vigorously back and forth, massage along several vertical (front-back) lines on the diagrams at once, for about three breaths, in and out.

- Similarly massage back and forth along the horizontal (left-right) lines on the diagrams.

- Next massage over the circles on the diagrams, working your fingers and hands in rapid circular motions.

◆ *Perform this entire procedure in the shower or when convenient. Even at seemingly low-stress times, stress receptors may need massaging nearly every day.*

◆ *Listen to your body. Active stress receptors in need of massage will call for attention, like an itch that needs scratching. Spend more time on those areas.*

See www.DrFrankKing.com for videos and more information about these and other HOT techniques.

HOT #6: FOREHEAD EMOTIONAL REFLEX POINTS TECHNIQUE

We all encounter daily stress, which negatively impacts health in more

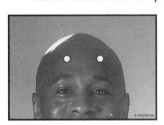

Forehead Emotional
Reflex Points

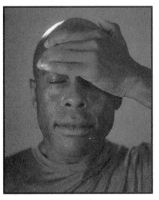

Forehead Massage

ways than we can imagine. In addition to the stress receptor massage described earlier, try this simple and effective technique to release stress and restore positive emotions and attitudes.

◆ *Place one hand against your forehead so that your palm and fingers cover the two emotional reflex points on the diagram.*

◆ *Very lightly tug the skin on your forehead in one direction. Hold your hand against the skin; do not massage. Many people find a gentle downward tug works best.*

◆ *Hold about four minutes while first thinking of the things that cause you stress. You may want to re-imagine peaceful and life-giving outcomes that will bring joy.*

◆ *You may feel a faint pulse over these points. If you do, and if the pulse on one side is different from the* other side, it often becomes synchronized as emotional tensions are released and resolved. Don't be surprised if you feel a strong emotional release with this technique. I've often seen that happen with my patients, and it is always good.

◆ Feel free to repeat this HOT as often as you like.

HOT #7: AURICULAR MASSAGE TECHNIQUE

The human body is so amazingly interconnected. Your ears, for example, contain a high concentration of acupuncture points connected by meridians to the major regions of your body. You can enhance your whole body's health with an auricular (ear) massage.

Imagine an upside-down human body in a fetal position, and that image gives you a good visualization of which body regions are enhanced by massaging related parts of your ear. For example, the ear lobe points connect to your head, the middle of your ear relates to your back and abdomen, and the upper ear relates to your feet and legs curled up.

◆ Begin by stretching your ears outward, by tugging in as many directions as possible.
◆ Use one or two fingers – with your thumb stabilized behind the ear – to massage one small section

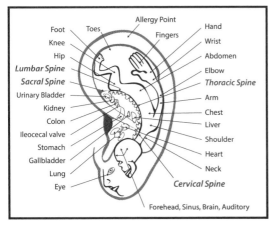

Foot Toes Allergy Point Hand
Knee Fingers Wrist
Hip Abdomen
Lumbar Spine Elbow
Sacral Spine *Thoracic Spine*
Urinary Bladder Arm
Kidney Chest
Colon Liver
Ileocecal valve Shoulder
Stomach Heart
Gallbladder Neck
Lung *Cervical Spine*
Eye
Forehead, Sinus, Brain, Auditory

Ear Massage Points

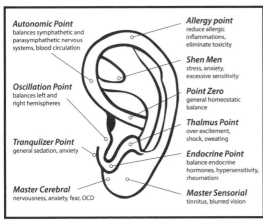

Autonomic Point
balances symphathetic and
parasymphathetic nervous
systems, blood circulation

Oscillation Point
balances left and
right hemispheres

Tranqulizer Point
general sedation, anxiety

Master Cerebral
nervousness, anxiety, fear, OCD

Allergy point
reduce allergic
inflammations,
eliminate toxicity

Shen Men
stress, anxiety,
excessive sensitivity

Point Zero
general homeostatic
balance

Thalmus Point
over excitement,
shock, sweating

Endocrine Point
balance endocrine
hormones, hypersensitivity,
rheumatism

Master Sensorial
tinnitus, blurred vision

For enhanced health benefits, massage these
acupuncture master points

of your ear for 15 seconds to a minute.

◆ Rub deep enough to find tender areas but not cause uncomfortable pain. Use precision and slightly change your angle of massage, listening to your instincts, giving attention where needed. The points are tiny and precise; they may be tender in their cry for therapeutic attention.

◆ Search new sections of your ear for tiny, tender spots, and massage them for up to a minute. Small BB-sized knots may require special attention, indicating areas of imbalance.

◆ Continue until each part of your ear has been massaged. Spend more time on ear points that relate to areas of the body that are in need of healing. Repeat about three

WHAT'S SO WONDERFUL ABOUT the AURICULAR MASSAGE TECHNIQUE?

Auricular massage has always been, for me, a simple but powerful tool for the toughest cases. If one of my patients wasn't experiencing a healing breakthrough – even while tapping, drinking plenty of water and making positive changes in all Eight Essentials – I often found the answer in auricular massage. Those two ears on the sides of your head, with their extensive acupuncture points and powerful connections to your entire body's form and function, have more power than you might think to help awaken healing. Try auricular therapy that add to your breakthroughs in your Healing Revolution.

times weekly or as often as desired.

◆ For additional health benefits throughout your entire body, massage the regions that are defined in the acupuncture master points diagram.

◆ More detailed diagrams, articles and videos about this and other HOT techniques can be found at www.DrFrankKing.com.

◆ This health-enhancing massage can be done anywhere and anytime, for example, while waiting in traffic or speaking on the phone.

◆ Auricular massage can be fun for couples; try sharing it with your partner or healing buddy.

HOT #8: SPHINCTER OF ODDI MASSAGE TECHNIQUE

The sphincter of Oddi is a ring-like muscle that regulates the flow of bile and pancreatic enzymes into the intestine. A constricted flow of digestive fluids through the sphincter of Oddi causes a broad spectrum of problems including incomplete digestion, bloating, gas, fatigue and cramping. More serious problems associated with enzyme deficiency include arthritis and even cancer. Massage the sphincter of Oddi to improve your internal health.

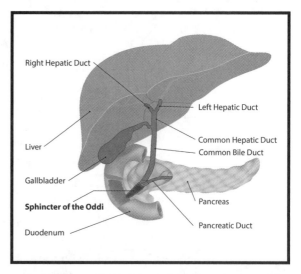

The Sphincter of Oddi delivers fluids from the liver, gall bladder and pancreas to the small intestine.

◆ To locate the sphincter of Oddi, go three finger-widths up from your belly button, and two finger-widths to the right of your midline.

◆ Press your fingers an inch or two into your gut. Move your fingers in different directions until you feel a tender area about the size of the tip of your little finger. Hold a comfortable pressure over the tender sphincter

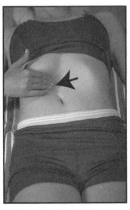

for 30 seconds. You may hear it gurgle as the sphincter of Oddi tension is released. Repeat until you hear no more gurgles.

◆ *Next, press the sphincter to your right and hold for 30 seconds. Repeat until you hear no more gurgles.*

◆ *Alternately, press it to the right and slightly up, or to the right and slightly down. Repeat until you hear no more gurgles. Repeat as often as needed.*

Sphincter of Oddi Massage

See www.DrFrankKing.com for videos and more helpful information about this and other HOT techniques.

WHAT'S SO AMAZING ABOUT the SPHINCTER OF ODDI MASSAGE TECHNIQUE?

The sphincter of Oddi is the great liberator. When functioning normally, it allows the digestive fluids from the liver, gall bladder and pancreas to do their wonder-working magic on your food. That in turn causes healthy enzymes to circulate throughout your body like happy little custodians, cleaning up your internal functions and preparing them for healthy service. A cramped, constricted sphincter of Oddi drastically reduces the flow of healthy enzymes. You could buy enzyme supplements in capsule form at the store, but they wouldn't be nearly as effective as those that flow naturally through the sphincter of Oddi. Allow your sphincter of Oddi to liberate your digestive health with this powerful HOT technique.

HOT #9: ILEOCECAL VALVE MASSAGE TECHNIQUE

Ileocecal valve problems affect 70 to 80 percent of the population. These disorders are the most common cause of autointoxification, which occurs when the body absorbs toxins from the bowel.

The ileocecal valve separates the small intestine from the large intestine. Its purpose is to prevent material from flowing backward into the small intestine. Think of it this way: The small intestine is like the kitchen in your

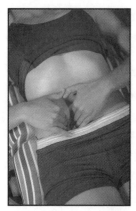

Ileocecal Valve Massage

house, digesting food and absorbing nutrients into your body. The large intestine is like your septic system, handling the nasty waste products. A malfunctioning ileocecal valve spasms and gets stuck open, like a broken valve that allows sewage to back up into your kitchen. You don't need that kind of problem in your gut!

Moreover, the ileocecal valve may be the secret for identifying your perfect diet. How? Because the ileocecal valve becomes irritated and inflamed with food allergies, toxicities and intolerances. Feel your valve periodically. If it is sensitive, note what foods you have eaten over the past 4 to 16 hours and try to make appropriate dietary adjustments. This will eventually lead you to discover your perfect diet.

Eating too much roughage can actually irritate the ileocecal valve. If ileocecal valve tenderness persists, and if your diet contains a large quantity of roughage such as raw fruits, vegetables, bran, popcorn, nuts or seeds, you may need to change your diet.

Here is how you can massage the ileocecal valve to relieve intestinal discomfort and to aid in digestive flow.

- ◆ *Lie on your back.*
- ◆ *Press firmly to locate a golf ball-sized lump in a tender depression, about one-third the way from the inside bump of your right hip bone to your belly button. This is the ileocecal valve.*
- ◆ *Press down firmly with the flat*

WHAT'S SO GREAT ABOUT the ILEOCECAL VALVE MASSAGE TECHNIQUE?

Whenever one of my patients had a zinc or vitamin C deficiency, I would massage the ileocecal valve. Tests would then show a fast increase in the deficient nutrient. Toxic waste from the large intestine is a thief when it backs up into the small intestine, robbing your body of essential immunonutrients including vitamins A, C, E, zinc and more. It poisons your gut, leading to bladder, stomach and reproductive problems. I've even had patients with chronic low-back pain that was relieved by this simple technique. Help your ileocecal valve function normally and keep the waste products flowing toward the sewage treatment plant – not back into the kitchen – with this simple technique. Monitoring your ileocecal valve will also help you discover your perfect diet.

surface of your fingers and hold for about 30 seconds. You may hear a gurgle or two.
- Repeat until you hear no more gurgles.
- Next move the valve slightly toward your midline and hold for about 30 seconds.
- If your ileocecal valve is irritated, it will be tender.
- You will hear a gurgling as it resets itself.
- Try pushing the valve in different directions: to the right, up and down. Hold each for 30 seconds. Repeat until you hear no more gurgles.
- If tender, massage two to three times a day: before getting up in the morning, after going to bed, or before each meal. You may experience tenderness for the first couple weeks until the valve's health and function is improved.
- Make positive dietary changes and reduce roughage, as needed, to reduce ileocecal valve tenderness. Homeopathic remedies and liquid chlorophyll may also help relieve tenderness.

Warning: See your doctor if you have had – or suspect – problems with your appendix, if you have a slight fever, or if tenderness persists.

HOT #10: KEEP YOUR SPINE IN LINE TECHNIQUES

The spine is like the circuit breaker for your neural communications. It houses the control network for every organ, gland, muscle and cell in your body. Unfortunately, many people suffer in many ways because their spines get out of shape and lose flexibility. Spinal dysfunction causes nerve interferences that can negatively impact the body in many ways. This problem is so pervasive that if you don't have spinal interferences, you are in a minority of the population. These simple and effective techniques will help maximize your overall health. Don't worry if you hear small popping sounds as you stretch your vertebrae.

▶ Super Spine Massage

This technique works and feels best with the help of a healing buddy, although you may be able to reach your neck and lower back yourself. Consider purchasing a body cushion or massage table that will comfortably

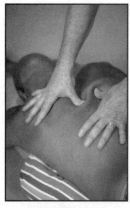

Super Spine

support your body, cradle your head and keep your neck and back straight while you are massaged.

◆ *Lie face-down on a bed, couch, floor or comfortable surface with your healing buddy beside you.*
◆ *Your healing buddy will use a combination of contacts including fingertips, thumbs, knuckles and the base of the hand beside each vertebrae.*
◆ *Your healing buddy will make small, deep, twisting, circular motions for 15 seconds or more on the deep, intrinsic muscles of the spine. The spine contains a complex network of muscles, so give each area as much massage as needed.*

◆ *Massage the entire spine, concentrating on tight and tender muscles.*

◆ *After massaging, apply pressure with fingers or thumbs to the tender areas for about 30 seconds each.*

◆ *To enhance health and healing in problem areas, finish with firm fingertip tapping on associated acupuncture points to the left and right of sore vertebrae (see diagram for those points). Tap with all fingers together for up to one minute. Tapping can be as effective as acupuncture treatment.*

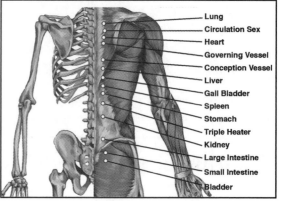

Associated Acupuncture Points

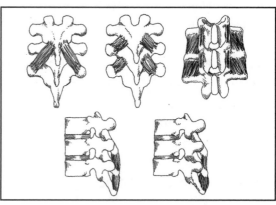

A complex network of muscles ties the vertebrae together, necessitating deep massage therapy.

Diagram used with permission of I.C.A.K.-USA©:
David S. Walther, *Applied Kinesiology; Synopsis 2nd Edition*
(Shawnee Mission, KS: Triad of Health Publishing, Inc., 2000), p. 72.

Related to this, you can buy a natural bristle, long-handled body brush to give yourself a dry brush back massage. Obey your instincts, massaging the areas that cry out for the most attention. (See page 127 for more information about Dry Brush Massage.)

▶ Spine: Arching ("Cat Stretch")

- Get on your hands and knees with your back parallel to the floor.
- Arch your back up toward the sky like a cat, comfortably stretching your vertebrae.
- Next, drop your belly toward the floor while lifting your chin up as high as you comfortably can, feeling your spine stretch.
- Repeat three or more times, until your spine feels well-stretched.

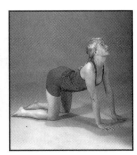

Spine: Arching Up   *Spine: Arching Down*

▶ Spine: Buttocks up and Belly Down

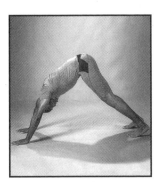
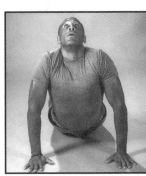

Spine: Buttocks Up   *Spine: Belly Down*

- Get in a push-up position with your hands and feet on the ground and your body parallel to the floor.
- Walk your feet up toward your head, while lifting your buttocks as high as you can, feeling your spine stretch.
- Next, walk your hands forward and drop your belly and arch your spine toward the floor, while lifting your chin up as high as you comfortably can, feeling your spine stretch.
- Repeat three or more times, until your spine feels well-stretched.

▶ Spinal Twist

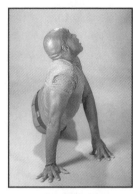

◆ *Get in a push-up position with your hands and feet on the ground and your body parallel to the floor. If necessary, rest your knees on the floor.*

◆ *Twist your hips, shoulders and head to the left, keeping your hands and feet on the floor while feeling the twisting action throughout your spine.*

◆ *Next, twist your hips, shoulders and head to the right while feeling the twisting action throughout your spine.*

Spinal Twist

◆ *Repeat three or more times, until your spine feels well-stretched.*

▶ Spine Roll

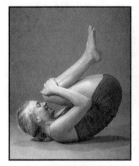

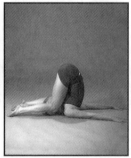

The Spine Roll improves flexibility, massages the spine and increases lymphatic circulation. Your whole body will feel better when your back is loosened and strengthened by the Spine Roll.

Spine Roll   *Spine Roll Advanced*

CAUTION: If you have health issues or are at risk of injury, consult with your healthcare practitioner before doing these exercises. Never force a motion if you experience pain.

◆ *Do this technique on a soft mat, comfortable carpet or rug.*

◆ *Lie on your back and draw your knees up to your chest with your hands. Hug your knees and begin a gentle rocking motion, rolling up and down your spine on the cushioned floor.*

◆ *Rock up and down, rolling your spine on the floor. Repeat five or more times, until your spine feels well-stretched.*

◆ *Roll further toward your head, resting on your shoulders and neck, eventually allowing your bent legs to dangle beside your head.* ***Do not attempt this if you have spinal pain or injury.***

- *Alternately, straighten your legs up in the air while making your spine as straight and vertical as possible, propping your hands against your back with your elbows on the floor.*

HOT #11: MUSCLE AND JOINT MASSAGE TECHNIQUE

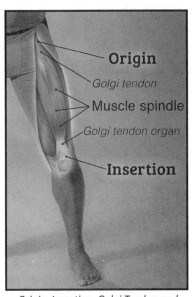

Origin

Golgi tendon

Muscle spindle

Golgi tendon organ

Insertion

Origin, Insertion, Golgi Tendon and Muscle Spindle Cells (the diagram shows the quadriceps muscles, although this HOT applies to all muscles)

Aerobics and weight training injuries have increased over 173 percent in recent years. One in five emergency room visits in the United States are the result of sports and exercise-induced injuries, according to the Centers for Disease Control.[117] Thankfully, the muscle and joint massage helps relieve pain, improve performance and prevent injury to muscles and joints. Proactively care for your muscles and joints by identifying tenderness, which is an indication of micro-trauma.

- *Use your fingertips to seek tender areas and massage the **origin and insertion** (the beginning and end) of muscles. Rub the tender areas firmly in a brisk, circular*

---

117   *Hidden Exercise Hazards Exposed: Are You Next?* www.maximizedliving.com/Home/MaximizedLivingBlog/ tabid/772/ Article/559/hidden-exercise-hazards-exposed-are-you-next.aspx (January 2014).

Here's a story I've heard too many times: "I got excited about a new exercise program. I worked like a dog to lose my first 10 pounds. Then I got this darn injury, so now I'm giving it all up." While some people strain like crazy to get off the ground with one exercise, you can soar up to the sky by working smarter, not harder, in all Eight Essentials of life. You also have a tool for avoiding future injury. After you exercise, give yourself a simple examination. Let your fingers do the walking, as you literally get in touch with your muscles. Probe your legs, arms and torso for tender spots. Ask your healing buddy for help with muscles you cannot reach. Proactively discover problems waiting to happen. Then nip future injuries in the bud with this muscle massage technique. Be aware of these tender areas and work on them, which will greatly minimize the chance of injury. Can you imagine all the time, money and suffering you have saved by not becoming an exercise-injury statistic?

motion, where the tendon is anchored into the bone.

• *Use your fingertips or palms to massage the **Golgi tendon**. Massage by pressing along the tendon and toward the middle (the "belly") of the muscle, away from the origin and insertion points. Repeat five to seven times. Massaging this area strengthens the attachments between muscle and tendon.*

♦ *Use the fingertips on both hands to massage the **muscle spindle cells**, which are sensory nerves in the belly of the muscle. Start with the fingers of both hands together at the center of the muscle. Press firmly and separate your fingers along the length of the muscle, toward the origin and insertion. Repeat five to seven times. This massage strengthens muscle function. See **www.DrFrankKing.com** for videos and more helpful information about this and other HOT techniques.*

HOT #12: RAGLAND'S TEST FOR ADRENAL FATIGUE

Fatigue, memory loss, foggy thinking and lack of enthusiasm, ambition and motivation are all common signs of adrenal fatigue. The Ragland's Test is a simple test for adrenal fatigue. All you need is a blood pressure cuff (the kind that goes on your upper arm), available online or locally from most drug stores. An automated cuff is by far the simplest, especially if you are not comfortable manually pumping up the pressure and listening through a stethoscope.

- *Place the automated cuff firmly on your upper arm.*
- *Lie on your back for four to five minutes.*
- *Press the button to activate the cuff, then take note of the top (systolic) number on the gauge.*
- ***CAUTION: Have someone assist you, or hold onto a railing for the next step, if you are prone to dizziness or passing out.***
- *After the cuff is deflated, activate the cuff again and immediately stand up. Note the top number.*
- *Your systolic pressure (the top number) should rise from 5 to 10 points when you stand up. A lower number is a sign of adrenal fatigue. The lower your systolic number drops, the more your adrenals are fatigued.*

WHAT'S SO SPECIAL ABOUT RAGLAND'S TEST?

Stress, low-grade inflammation, allergies and toxicities all contribute to adrenal fatigue, which can eventually lead to burnout. Many people never discover the cause of their burnout and fatigue. Over 80 percent of my patients had adrenal issues, as diagnosed by the Ragland's Test. This simple, diagnostic tool does not require the expense and trouble of doctor's visits and insurance forms. Moreover, doctors rarely perform this safe and effective test for adrenal fatigue. Thankfully, the causes of adrenal fatigue can be addressed by making natural lifestyle changes in the Eight Essentials of life.

My recommendations to patients with adrenal fatigue include: 1) take our Whole Person Appraisal at www.DrFrankKing.com, with a special focus on the mind-body section to identify root causes of stress, 2) practice all Eight Essentials to build up your adrenals, 3) take supplements such as vitamin C, pentatonic acid, licorice root, ginseng, gynostemma, and adrenal extract, and 4) seek professional medical help if you are unable to correct the problem. I also invite you to contact me through my website for a network of qualified doctors who use natural therapies that will help you succeed in the Healing Revolution.

TIP is great to use in conjunction with each one of these HOT techniques, especially if you encounter difficulties or obstacles. For example, tap to statements like, "I am confident and able to succeed with this HOT. I am becoming whole and healthy with the help of this HOT. I am confident and able to share this Hands On Technique with others."

Sharing with others is a sure sign that you are becoming fully engaged in the Healing Revolution. Teachers will tell you that their knowledge and love for a topic increases dramatically when they teach it to others. The same is true with these healing tools. I have seen so many people's healing increase exponentially when they began sharing what they learned with others.

Are you as excited about these Hands On Techniques as I am? Many of my patients have found health, healing and wholeness through these simple but very effective techniques … and so can you! I encourage you to visit www.DrFrankKing.com for free videos and more information about HOTs and many other life-affirming techniques. Tell me about your journey to wholeness. Connect with us through our social media sites.[118]

Begin your Healing Revolution today. Take back your health! Awaken the healing power within you!

118   See www.facebook.com/kingbionaturalmedicine, twitter.com/KingBiodotcom and LinkedIn: Dr. Frank King.

SELF-EVALUATION
TOP 12 CHANGES

Review your Self-Evaluations from the other Eight Essentials. List here or in your Health Journal the top 12 changes that you'd like to make. Some changes may be quick and easy; others may take some time.

My Life-Destroying Choices	My Life-Affirming Choices
1	1
2	2
3	3
4	4
5	5
6	6
7	7
8	8
9	9
10	10
11	11
12	12

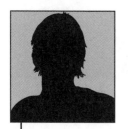

One Girl's Story:
Putting the Earth Together

A doctor I knew had a five-year-old girl who wanted to play with her daddy. Unfortunately, the father was exhausted from a long day at work. All he wanted was a few minutes of shut-eye. So he grabbed a *Life* magazine and tore out a full-page photo of the earth that had been taken from outer space.

"What are you doing, Daddy?" she asked, as he tore the picture into about 30 pieces.

"I'm making a puzzle for you, sweetheart," he said. "See if you can put all these pieces back together. When you finish, you'll have a complete picture of the world."

The father gave her the pieces and some clear tape. Then he sunk back into his easy chair. With all the dark space and blue earth in that picture, he figured it would take her quite a while to put it all back together.

He was just drifting off into orbit around his own distant galaxy when suddenly he was jerked back to consciousness.

"Hey Daddy. Look at this!"

The man took a deep breath and sat up to see a big, bright smile on the girl's face. On the coffee table was the magazine page, perfectly assembled.

"Wow!" said the father. "You put that together so fast. And it looks great. How did you do it so quickly?"

"Let me show you." She flipped the puzzle over. "You see ... there's a picture of a man on the back side."

She was right. It was obvious that the human figure was much simpler to assemble than the world.

"I just put the man together," she said. "When I turned it over, the world was back together too."

She put the man together and the world took care of itself.

That is a brilliant illustration of the Healing Revolution. We are stewards of ourselves, as well as stewards of the world. We are interconnected, finding connectedness with each other as well as with the world, as outlined in both the Nature and Relationships chapters. Our paths intersect in the ground that bears our food, upon which we bear our children.

As each one of us becomes more whole, we are able to think more whole, act more whole, and take care of the earth in a more holistic manner.

Let us live out that beautiful vision that this little girl stated so perfectly. As we naturally put ourselves back together, the earth will *naturally* take care of itself.

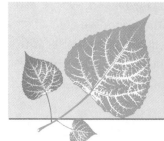

YOUR STORY: CHOOSE YOUR OWN ENDING

*It was the best of times, it was the worst of times, it
was the age of wisdom, it was the age of foolishness, it
was the epoch of belief, it was the epoch of incredulity,
it was the season of Light, it was the season of
Darkness, it was the spring of hope, it was the winter
of despair, we had everything before us, we had
nothing before us, we were all going direct to Heaven,
we were all going direct the other way.*

– Charles Dickens, "A Tale of Two Cities"

Once upon a time people lived close to the earth. They grew their food from their own soil. They apprenticed their kids in the fields and workshops. Their life cycles followed the natural rhythms of sun and season. Hearts of horse and master beat in synch. Tribes huddled together for warmth and protection. Healers shared wisdom they had received from previous generations.

This was normal life for thousands of years until one day the "experts" had an innovative idea.

"Hey!" they said. "Let's bulldoze all these unsanitary farms and replace them with nice, clean factories that will grind up food and put it in tidy boxes. We'll send the kids to institutions to learn. We'll send sick people to institutions to get better. We'll put institutions in charge of our laws and money. Experts will make all of our decisions so we'll have nothing to worry about. We'll invent light bulbs so everyone can work longer days, even in the wintertime! We may even give workers something called a 'vacation' once each year as an incentive for them to work harder. And all this walking that people do … it's terribly old fashioned. We'll make square boxes on wheels for whooshing people around. When people get home from work totally exhausted, they'll eat food out of boxes in front of another kind of box that ... well, it's difficult to explain. Then they'll fall asleep in a box-like room, until another little box makes an irritating noise to interrupt their dreams."

Forgive me if this sounds naïve, but ... is life really that much better now that we are "civilized"? Have the so-called "experts" forgotten what we already know from our rich, natural, genetic heritage? Sure, this is the "best of times" when you think of the plagues and common sicknesses that have been contained by sanitation. But does that really outweigh the pandemic of chronic illnesses and human suffering that modernity has impressed upon us? Hmm ...

No, I am not suggesting that we go back in time, but my simple observations tell me that people are happier and healthier when they live more simply and in tune with the natural ways of life. By doing so, we can wisely have the best of both worlds. We can embrace the positive aspects of modernity while never forgetting our natural healing abilities. There has never been a greater moment in time to awaken the Healing Revolution within each one of us.

BICYCLING AT THE AGE OF 100?

As mentioned earlier, we stand at the crossroads. One road leads to a long and happy life; the other to avoidable chronic disease and untimely death. Dr. Walter Bortz of Stanford University, author of *The Roadmap to 100*, describes two primary destinations for those of us who are journeying into the 21st century. A number of people will live longer and healthier, while many others will live shorter and sicker lives. The gulf between these two paths is widening.

Dr. Bortz suggests several lifestyle choices that will add years to your life (although the benefits in years are obviously not promises but potentials):

> *There is no simpler, more effective treatment to restore health and quality of life than the cure Mother Nature provides through natural living.*
>
> **– Dr. Paul C. Bragg**

◆ *Eat more fruits, vegetables and whole foods (add 5 years to your life)*
◆ *Exercise five days a week (add 2 to 4 years)*

- *Reduce stress (add up to 6 years)*
- *Get a hobby (add 2 years)*
- *Take a regular vacation (add 1 to 2 years)*
- *Sleep eight hours nightly (add 2 years)*
- *Have a healthy sex life (add 3 to 5 years)*
- *Floss your teeth to remove harmful bacteria (add 6 years)*

Research also establishes the benefits of these additional lifestyle habits:

- *Sit less than three hours a day (add 2 years to your life)*
- *Watch less than two hours of television per day (add 1.38 years)*[119]

Remarkably, that all adds up to about *35 extra years of life* (no guarantees, of course). More importantly, positive choices in all Eight Essentials of life will improve your chances of attaining a high *quality of life*. Our lifespan need not exceed our *health-span*.

"A hundred years is securely established as the human potential," says Dr. Bortz. (Although I would add, "Why stop at one hundred?") If you have any questions about Dr. Bortz practicing what he preaches, he ran his 40th marathon … at the age of 80.[120] Jeanne Louise Calment of Arles, France, who died at 122 was still riding her bicycle at the age of 100.

People like that really get me excited about growing old. This is what the Healing Revolution is all about. Too many people expect to live to 60 or 70 because that's when their parents died. Reset your mindset. Reimagine your future and set higher goals. See yourself living like Moses of the Bible whose body was vigorous and eyes were not dim when he his life ended at the age of 120.[121]

---

119   Katzmarzyk PT, Lee I-M, op cit.

120   Walter M. Bortz II and Randall Stickrod, *The Roadmap to 100: The Breakthrough Science of Living a Long and Healthy Life* (New York: Palgrave Macmillan, 2010); and *Active Over 50*, Spring Issue 2010, www.activeover50.com\issuses\AO50_Spring_10_LR.pdf (January 2014).

121   Deuteronomy 34:7.

ROGER: THE REST OF THE STORY

Remember the story of Roger, the psychologist who was so depressed that he could barely function? (page 61) Roger was so focused on his patients' problems that he actually became their problems. As mentioned earlier, Roger was finally liberated with the aid of TIP (Tap Into Potential).

But that is only part of the story. I explained to Roger the interconnectedness of the Eight Essentials of life, and how health is enhanced by making small, positive changes in all eight areas.

Well, Roger already knew that he was a junk food junkie, so he tried reaching for delicious, real foods when his stomach called out for attention. As he did so, his appetite for fake, chemically-enhanced snacks began to fade. He cultivated a taste for life-giving water instead of diet sodas. He passionately embraced my recommendation to walk more and drive less.

One memorable experience happened early in his journey to wholeness.

"I saw these shaggy-looking guys playing Frisbee in the city park yesterday," he told me, "and out of the blue, they tossed the Frisbee my way."

"That's great!" I said with a laugh. "How did it go?"

Roger looked sheepish. "Not so good. I never played Frisbee before." I could hear the embarrassment in his voice. "I tried to catch that Frisbee, but it just hit my body with a thud and fell to the ground. Then I attempted to throw it back, but it just flopped and went nowhere. I might as well have been tossing a dead cat."

"Well, don't let it bother you, Roger. At least you tried."

"Yeah," he said with a grin. "Actually, they showed me how to hold it, how to wind my arm up like a spring and throw it so it spins. I made a few decent throws, although my aim was terrible. Still, they invited me to come back and play Frisbee again. They're out there tossing it around nearly every day, just about the time I get off work."

"Good for you, Roger." I heaped as much encouragement on Roger as I possibly could. It was so exciting for me to see him taking small, positive steps with all Eight Essentials.

Back when Roger was in the depths of depression, he spent most of his time indoors under artificial lighting, working at his desk in front of a computer. He complained about having no energy and not being able to sleep well. He was depressed. He'd sit inside and watch TV each night. He was cut off from the natural joys of real life, as if he were a zombie.

That's why I was so thrilled to see him take so many small steps in different areas of life. He began to commune with nature. He breathed deep of vitamin "O" and was seen by Doctor Sunshine. Soon he was sleeping deeper and feeling better rested. He had much more energy and enthusiasm for life. He practiced tapping and other healing techniques that I showed him.

Roger's relationships even improved. He made friends with the shaggy dudes from the park. He got to be pretty darn good at playing Frisbee. Surprisingly, Roger didn't even have to work hard to see positive results. The small changes he made in all Eight Essentials multiplied exponentially, allowing him to see tremendous overall results. Roger was working smarter, not harder.

When I last saw Roger, he had made awesome life-affirming choices in all Eight Essentials. Moreover, his private practice that was in danger of going belly-up because of his depression had actually tripled. Roger was prospering in nearly every way possible. That's the beauty of the Healing Revolution.

REVISITING CAROL'S STORY

Hopefully you are getting REALLY EXCITED to discover practical ways of implementing the Healing Revolution in all Eight Essential areas of your life. To help you do so, let's revisit Carol's story from page 134. She's the woman who came into our clinic for help with a chronic hip problem ... whose Healing Revolution exploded miraculously into every corner of her life.

Carol became serious enough at that critical transition in her life to attend 10-weeks of classroom sessions that we provided on Monday nights. She made an huge effort to participate, even after long days at work, in rain and snow and all kinds of weather. She also totally invested herself in life-affirming changes in all Eight Essentials of life. We revisit her story here at the end of the book to inspire you, so you can see how Carol did it. She's a regular person, just like you and me. If she can do it, so can you!

In the following chart, I'll fill in more of her details about her life. You'll see how she had a full assortment of problems that were all interconnected. That's no surprise, since we are whole beings and all of our systems are

CAROL'S TRANSFORMATION

ESSENTIAL	VICTIM	- TO -	VICTOR
Engaging the Power of the Human Spirit	She was 30 to 40 pounds overweight, which depressed her. She was chronically fatigued, lethargic and she had a low self-image.	Inspired by quick chiropractic results, Carol gained the DESIRE to change. She BELIEVED that change was possible and powerful.	Her spirit was lifted to a whole new dimension. Her energy and enthusiasm for life blossomed. She was happier, healthier and had a great self-image.
Eat real food	She tried every possible diet, while not being able to give up sweets. High blood sugar and bromine was causing thyroid and adrenal problems.	She learned about the harmful effects of bromine in white flour and pastries, and stopped eating them. She also stopped putting bromine in the hot tub.	Carol loved eating healthy food. She was passionate about helping others with good nutrition. She replaced refined salt with sea salt and a natural iodine supplement.
Drink Real Water	Her weight fluctuated by as much as five pounds in a day, due to water retention. She drank diet soda and city water.	She learned about the harms of diet soda, and the problems with chlorine and fluoride in city water.	She loved drinking spring water, and lots of it. She had no more water retention problems.
Functional Fitness	She first came to my office because of chronic hip pain. This was related to adrenal fatigue and her sedentary lifestyle choices.	She came alive, due to her changed diet and daily ET exercises.	Carol felt GREAT about her beautiful arms, legs and face, no longer buried under cellulite. She loved biking and walking, alone and with friends.
Super-natural sleep	She stayed up late watching TV and didn't usually sleep enough.	She learned about the value of 8 to 9 hours of quality sleep.	She enjoyed full nights of restful sleep, awaking refreshed in the morning.
Relate with nature	She rarely got outdoors. Nature was not important to her. She'd rather watch soap operas.	She spent less time watching TV and more time going for walks and gardening in the backyard.	Quiet times in nature became sacred times for Carol. She loved the fresh air and sunshine.
Relationships	Her low self-image and poor health contributed to an unhealthy marriage.	She learned how whole body-mind health is related to relationships.	She became confident in her self-image, and fulfilled in her marriage and friendships.
Hands On Techniques	She was lethargic and had little energy to try and improve her condition.	Simple home tests and MRT helped us identify thyroid and adrenal problems. TIP helped her make positive changes.	Hands On Techniques became a regular part of Carol's new, healthy life. Her future never looked so bright.

interconnected. Her healing, therefore, was similarly united and holistic. In this chart, you'll see how Carol made a miraculous transformation from victim to victor.

Carol became so passionate about health that – like a missionary – she converted many friends and family to the Healing Revolution. She ended up referring at least one new patient to our clinic, each and every month!

Carol's cocoon-to-butterfly story can be your story as well. I have seen many so-called "incurable" conditions overcome in the Healing Revolution. Expect dramatic results as you awaken the healing power within you.

Are you ready for the most incredible, powerful, exciting time of your life, greater than you can ever hope, dream or imagine?!?

COME ON IN, THE WATER'S FINE!

> Life is a river, always flowing
>
> – Mahatma Gandhi

My oldest son Frankie knows the bottom of the Nolichucky River better than anybody I know. We kayaked the rapids together when he was a kid, and I fished him out more times than I can recall. The Nolichucky River Gorge on the Tennessee-North Carolina border is quite a thrill, with dozens of extreme rapids carved into a stunning, 3,000-foot deep gorge. Sometimes Frankie and I would take a break from kayaking to jump off a tall railroad bridge, or ride a natural water-slide over a waterfall so high that we barely had enough breath to last until we popped like corks back to the surface of the deep water below.

If you fall out of your watercraft in the middle of rapids, the key to survival is simply to go with the flow. People who fight the flow and try to stand or brace themselves in a difficult spot have drowned when a foot or leg got caught in the crevice of a rock. Going with the flow means keeping your feet downstream and letting your life jacket float you to safety. Once you know how to do it, falling out of the boat is so fun that you totally enjoy the ride.

That's a wonderful philosophy for life. The river of life will take you through some of the most gorgeous scenery you can imagine. But it will also carry you through some rough rapids, past snags and over waterfalls. Ride the rapids. Go with the flow. The challenges will make you stronger if you let them.

You will encounter some tempting forks in the river. Like the crossroads we discussed earlier, these forks lead far away from the natural, healthy flow of the river. These diversions lead to toxic and polluted swamps. Let the Eight Essentials be your map, your GPS and your guidebook to keep you in the life-giving flow of this scenic river of life.

Can you feel the flow? Rest back and float on your lifejacket. Let the waters carry you. Can you feel the warm sunlight on your face? Do you see the lazy willows swaying gently in the breeze? This delicious river carries you to new vistas and breathtaking scenery. Can you enjoy the ride?

Come on in, the water's fine!

This is the joy of living life to the fullest. This is not a self-help program or a list of tedious dos and don'ts. Don't struggle and strive like a "human doing."

Go with the flow!

Discover the joy of *being.*

Be a Human Being.

No need to stress when the water starts to churn. No need to worry about things that might never happen, or create problems that aren't there, when you can simply go with the flow. The rapids are just one part of this beautiful life. Imagine yourself downstream, beyond the rapids, saying, "Wow. What a ride!" You are stronger and better because of the rapids. You don't want to be like a wet towel that absorbs and holds problems. Be an unsinkable duck, bobbing jubilantly over all the churning waters of life.

Love life and live free. Enjoy the fulfillment of sharing this joy with the people around you. What can be better than that?

DESIRE, BELIEVE, BECOME

Your personal Healing Revolution begins with the tools in this book, which are designed to reset your vision for all you hope to be. You can reset your desire, your will, your beliefs, your faith and your ability to become healthy and whole.

Most people's approach to life and health is based on what is wrong with themselves.

"I got a membership at the gym," someone says, "because of *my fat thighs*."

"I hope my cancer doesn't come back."

"I can't get *my allergies* under control."

"It's just *my bad luck*," says another person. Or, "*My stupid decisions* are catching up with me."

"It's hell being old."

People personalize their deficits. They define themselves by their problems.

Imagine a man on a treadmill or a woman on a diet. Both can never reach their destination because they are constantly looking back at the person they despise. They are hopelessly tied to that old flawed self-image. They cannot see what lies ahead because they have never painted a picture of the person they could become. Without vision, people do perish.

Your destiny has nothing to do with the fat, sick, unfortunate and stupid person you once were.

You can shed that old image now.

Stand out in a field and scream and shout over that sick image, if that helps you.

Call that image out for being a liar. That sick image *is not you*!

Shed that image.

Kill that image.

Burn it.

Destroy it.

Mourn it, if you must.

Shed tears over that dead image of yourself.

Symbolically bury that dead image in the ground.

Cry your eyes out and let your tears water the grave of "your cancer," "your sickness," "your weight problem" or whatever "your deficit" might *have been*.

It is not yours anymore!

Shout it if you must: ***"THAT DEFICIT IS NOT MINE ANYMORE!"***

That deficit is now dead.

Turn your back on it.

Walk away from it.

Mention that deficit's name *no more*.

Forever leave behind the person you once were.

Now turn to discover the new you.

Take a deep, cleansing breath.

A heavy burden has fallen from your shoulders.

Replace it with a new, healthy picture of who you are to become.

Nothing destroys the old negative images as powerfully as when you replace them with bright, new, visions of life, health and wholeness.

You are now free to define your destiny.

You are now free to release and experience the healing power that is within you.

DESIRE.   What do you desire? Your passionate desire for a life-giving destiny will draw you positively forward like an irresistible magnet. Use TIP to help awaken your desire for abundant life.

BELIEVE.   Have faith in the new person that you are becoming. YOU CAN BE IT! Never doubt that fact. Use TIP to awaken positive, healthy beliefs in your heart and mind. Ask your Higher Power for help and strength beyond your abilities. Believe until you Become.

BECOME.   You will become what you believe – it's just that simple. Say to yourself, "I AM whole. I AM healthy. I AM complete. I AM experiencing peace, joy, love and all good things." Use TIP to reinforce your new self-image.

Put your new vision and destiny in black and white: Write it down in your Health Journal or here in this book. Set high goals for yourself, expecting real and powerful transformation, allowing this new image to permeate your entire being and saturate your body, mind and spirit. Do not shrink your world by only believing the limited things that science can validate in a laboratory, or you will be stuck in the age of flat earth medicine.

GOODBYE, FLAT EARTH MEDICINE

Imagine meeting the first explorers who just returned from sailing around the world.

"The world isn't flat," they exclaimed. "We followed the sun all the way around the globe, chasing it from sea to sea."

"And you never fell off the edge of the earth?" the people wondered in amazement.

"We never fell off, because there is no edge! The earth is round!"

Unfortunately there were no photographs or satellite maps to validate the journey, so the people on the wharf fell into a heated debate. They created such a ruckus that soon everyone from beggars to princes had gathered to participate.

"It can't be true," said a fishmonger, his arms folded across his thick chest.

"My granddad went out and he never returned. Fell off the edge of the earth, he did."

"How do you know if nobody saw him?" asked one of the sailors.

"He fell off, he did," repeated the fishmonger.

"Round earth? Bah!" said a politician with disgust. "As if people could walk upside-down on the other side."

"They'd fall straight up into the air," someone said with a laugh.

"It's preposterous!"

An ugly argument broke out between the flat- and round-earth opponents. Men and women shook their fists and jeered at each other.

At the edge of the crowd, a little girl in a dirty white smock tugged quietly on the sleeve of one of the dark-skinned sailors. The thick man knelt down on the weathered boards so he could hear what the girl had to say.

"Hey Mister," she said. Her blue eyes were wide and bright, as if to match the intensity of the brilliant Atlantic sea and sun. "Is it true what you said? Did you really sail all the way around the world?"

A huge smile crossed the swarthy man's face, but he didn't say a word. He simply nodded and winked his eye.

The little girl gave that seasoned sailor a great, big hug. "I knew it," she said, her bright eyes glistening with moisture. "My father is coming back home!"

Listen to those who have taken the journey.

The days of flat earth medicine are over.

Welcome to the Healing Revolution.

Desire.
Believe.
Become.

AUTHOR'S AUTOBIOGRAPHY:
DR. FRANK KING

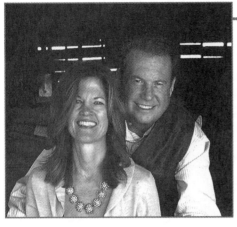

When I was five years old, I was so weak and scrawny that the doctors thought I might have leukemia. In desperation, my parents took me to a natural healer named Dr. Wickenham who lived in a run-down trailer park. "Dr. Wicked Hand," as my friends called him, discovered that I had serious food allergies. I changed my diet and was soon running with the other kids and working hard on my father's farm on the Ohio-Pennsylvania border.

People said my dad did the work of 10 men. After the Great Depression, he bought three-acres of land on the Ohio-Pennsylvania border where he built a gas station. He eventually expanded his holdings to include guest cabins, motel, bar, restaurant, bakery, barns, sheds and a 450-acre farm. He bulldozed a 30-acre lake out of a swamp and built a gorgeous 5,200 square foot home. In that beautiful, rural setting, I loved catching frogs and snakes, and raising anything from an injured owl to an alligator that we brought back from Florida. I enjoyed working as a veterinarian's assistant for several years. I learned to operate farm machinery, pump gas, change tires, change beds, serve meals, bartend, clear land, care for livestock and show cattle in competitions around the country. I liked dashing to the convenience store across the highway with my friends for junk food, until I met a peculiar man named Karl with a thick Eastern-European accent who taught me how to collect all different kinds of wild, edible plants.

I attended a rough Youngstown, Ohio, middle-high school that thickened my skin and showed me the best and worst sides of humanity. Boxing became my hobby and survival technique for about five years. Early in my boxing experiences, an injury sent me crashing to the floor, my spine exploding in pain. I could barely walk for weeks and several doctor's visits brought me no relief. My mother took me to a chiropractor. He treated my spine, muscles, acupuncture points, and even a valve in my intestine, and soon I was feeling better than ever. This experience heightened my interest in natural health.

As my dad got older, my family put me in charge of the farm since my older brothers were running the restaurant, motel and gas station. My passion for all things natural was growing by leaps and bounds, so I converted our operations to an organic, biodynamic farm in the early 1970s.

Meanwhile my enthusiasm for the healing arts also grew. I read everything I could about natural foods and health. I went to hear a crazy eighty-year-old man named Dr. Paul Bragg speak, and he dynamited my old-age stereotypes by lecturing on his head! A few years later, I was astounded to hear that he reportedly died from complications received from a surfing accident. These were my days of discovery as I learned how detrimental many aspects of the Industrial Revolution and the so-called advances of modern science and technology have been to human health. I began to see a need for another kind of revolution.

I still remember the day in 1975 when I decided to become a healer instead of a farmer. My life became a whirlwind of change that included chiropractic and naturopathic college. I obtained two degrees as Doctor of Chiropractic and Naturopathic Doctor. I established a natural health clinic that grew to include four doctors and 13 therapeutic staff.

People drove from miles around to visit our clinic that was located in the spacious house my father had built on our farm. We gained a reputation for catching people who were at the end of their ropes, whose challenging symptoms left other doctors scratching their heads. "Specializing in Difficult Cases" became the tag line on our business cards. Our new-patient evaluation was comprehensive, covering all the areas that came to be known as the Eight Essentials. We were passionate about finding all the root causes of illness, rather than simply treating the symptom. My experience with animals led me to help pet owners by giving chiropractic adjustments and natural remedies to dogs, cats, horses, buffalos and even chickens.

After all those years of seeing so many difficult cases, we developed new approaches to natural healthcare, including pure water-based homeopathic medicines, herbal nutritional extracts and new super-foods. I loved helping all the precious people in our clinic, but that busy practice left me no time to pursue my heart's passion of researching and developing natural, life-giving products and techniques. So in 1989 we established King

Bio, an FDA-registered company that researches, manufactures and sells natural products. Our brands include Dr. King's Natural Medicine, Safecare, SafeCareRx, Aquaflora, Natural Pet and Natural Vet.

In addition to being a practitioner in the healing arts, I'm a fourth-generation farmer. In 1985, I began raising bison as a healthier source of meat, eventually establishing Carolina Bison (www.carolinabison.com/). Our mission is to discover and promote healthier lifestyles by offering

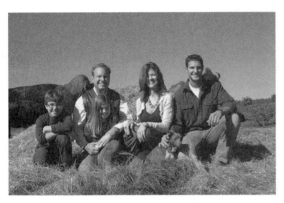

healthy meats and other wild super-foods that awaken our positive genetic expressions. We raise wild muscadine grapes, therapeutic herbs, elk, yak, Russian boar, wisent, watusi and camels for milk.

When we relocated to the Southern Appalachian Mountains, which contain the largest temperate rain forest in North America, we desired to take advantage of the natural biodiversity. The hearty environment of Western North Carolina has enabled us to research and develop a wide variety of wild, nutrient-rich and medicinal fruits, vegetables and herbs. My wife, Suzie, our children, and I live naturally on our farm in the Blue Ridge Mountains of Western North Carolina, enjoying everything from native muscadine grapes to camel's milk and bison steaks.

For more information about Dr. Frank King, see www.DrFrankKing.com.

Since 1989, *King Bio* has helped people find health, happiness and wholeness through *safe and natural*, pure water-based homeopathic and other natural medicines. Dr. King believes there are no diseases or conditions that your body cannot heal. He developed a complete line of natural medicines to activate the body's remarkable self-healing potential. See www.kingbio.com for more information.

KING BIO – NATURAL MEDICINES TO AWAKEN YOUR HEALING POTENTIAL

Dr. Frank King established Carolina Bison, one of the largest bison herds in the southeastern United States, in 1985. For more information, see www.carolinabison.com/.

Dr. Frank King started the Natural Medicine Institute (NMI), a 501(c)3 nonprofit to develop innovative educational programs and research using natural medicines and healing techniques as a basis for improved healthcare solutions.

Dr. King also established the Wild Food Foundation, a 501(c)3 nonprofit for the research and development of new, wild super-foods, sustainable organic agricultural methods and food production that awaken the roots of our healthy, genetic expressions, being mutually beneficial for humans, animals, plants and the environment.

 Tell us about your journey to health and wholeness at www.DrFrankKing.com, where you will find more helpful information about the Healing Revolution.

Connect and share with others in the Healing Revolution community at www.facebook.com/kingbionaturalmedicine, twitter.com/KingBiodotcom and *LinkedIn: Dr. Frank King*.